The Handbook of Hip & Knee Joint Replacement:

Through the Eyes of the Patient, Surgeon & Medical Team

The Handbook
of Hip & Knee
Joint Replacement:

Through the Eyes of the
Patient, Surgeon
& Medical Team

By

Ronald R. Hugate Jr., MD

and

Robert D. Holland, PMP

Table of Contents

Foreword by Dr. Ross Wilkins

Very often in considering decisions about an upcoming surgical intervention, patients can become intimidated, confused, or disorganized with their thoughts and decisions. This is due to the natural anxiety that patients may experience and the complex medical world through which they must navigate to make the right decisions for themselves. To most people, surgery is associated with negativity- losing one's consciousness, having to deal with pain, and significant physical and emotional stress. Dr. Hugate and Mr. Holland have collaborated to produce a very unique approach to answering the questions and guiding the decisions required when considering joint replacement. The knowledge they impart in this handbook will help to disarm the natural anxiety that patients may experience and make for a better overall experience and outcome.

Simply put, Dr. Hugate and Mr. Holland have developed a format for the conversation between the physician and the patient to assure that appropriate information is exchanged, explained, and understood. The end effect is that both patient and physician have significant understanding of the process and expected results. This is basically a "common sense" approach to major decisions that will affect the patient for the rest of their life. I encourage patient and physician alike to read this handbook and learn by its example. It sets a new standard for surgeon-patient communications.

Congratulations to the authors for this outstanding contribution.

Ross M. Wilkins, MD

Medical Director, Denver Clinic for Extremities at Risk

Founder and President, Limb Preservation Foundation

Dr. Hugate's Acknowledgements

I'd like to take a moment to acknowledge those who were instrumental in my personal development and in bringing this handbook to fruition.

Thanks to my many mentors who worked tirelessly to help make me the best surgeon and person I could be. It is said that mentors are individuals who turn their hindsight into your foresight. Dr. Vincent Pellegrini, Dr. Franklin Sim, Dr. David Goodspeed, Dr. James Holmes, and Dr. Ross Wilkins are among many who have selflessly donated their hindsight.

Thank you to my wonderful family for supporting me every step along the long and difficult road to becoming a surgeon. Without your support, love, and pride, I would certainly not have the privilege of doing what I do.

Thanks to Dr. Gianni Checa for contributing his expertise in anesthesiology to our handbook. He is one of only a handful of anesthesiologists whom I entrust with the care of my patients. He has distinguished himself through his extraordinary skill and bedside manner. Dr. Checa is not only an excellent anesthesiologist, he is a friend as well.

My gratitude also goes to Inger Brueckner, MSPT for lending her significant expertise to this handbook in a way that brings her subject to life for the reader. Physical therapy is as much about effectively interacting with patients as it is about technical excellence, and Inger is good at both.

Walter Buck PhD is both an Anatomist and friend. He volunteered to read and provide guidance on the anatomical descriptions and technical, rhetorical passages presented throughout the entire handbook and for that I am grateful. His skilled review has ensured the completeness and accuracy of this handbook for our readers.

Thank you to my patients for entrusting me with your care. There is no greater trust you can bestow upon another human being than that of your health. I am truly honored to be your doctor.

And finally, I would like to acknowledge and thank one of my patients and now coauthor, Robert Holland, PMP. Thank you for bringing the need for such a handbook to my attention, and for your tireless efforts in pushing this project forward. Capturing the attention of surgeons can be like herding cats! Robert was not only able to capture my attention with this idea, he also hoisted the project upon his shoulders and carried us to the finish line. For that, I am grateful.

Mr. Holland's Acknowledgements

Acknowledgements go to my wife, Vicki Holland, MBA, for her support, encouragement, and patronage throughout this project. Throughout the time Dr. Hugate and I toiled away on this manuscript, Vicki was working hard at her job, making ends meet for our family, pushing me to do better and work harder. Without her support this handbook would never have seen the light of day.

I also want to thank Francine Campone, EdD. Her wonderful insights, contributions, and comments throughout brought balance and perspective to our handbook and fairly represented the journey through hip replacement in a book coauthored by a knee replacement patient and an orthopedic surgeon.

Lastly, thanks to Dr. Hugate. His steady hands and quiet intelligence have guided me through some very hard times. He has healed me when I needed him and encouraged me when my determination flagged. You will be very lucky indeed if you find a surgeon like him.

How to Use This Handbook

Welcome to *The Handbook of Hip and Knee Replacement*. Among the strengths of our handbook are the various perspectives we bring to the table. This handbook has two coauthors and three contributors who lend their voices, opinions, and wisdom in various places throughout. Accordingly, we have made it very easy for you (the reader) to determine which writer is speaking.

The text of this handbook is broken down into the standard text and interposed commentary from our various contributors. Standard text will be preceded by a small photo of the author of that particular section and will be written in standard font. Commentary text will be preceded by small avatars (postage stamp pictures as shown below) for that particular comment. You will also notice that the font used in the comment text differs from that of the standard text as well. Comments are ended with a tilde-asterisk-tilde (~*~) so you know when the author (of whichever *chapter* you're reading) is speaking again.

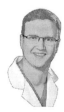 Here are the avatars for coauthor Ronald R. Hugate Jr., MD. Dr. Hugate is an orthopedic surgeon who specializes in joint replacements and treating complex orthopedic problems. Throughout the text, Dr. Hugate comments often, so we'll use two avatars for him.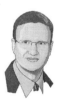

 This is avatar represents Robert Holland, PMP. Robert is also a coauthor of this handbook. He brings perspective as a patient who has received two total knee replacements.

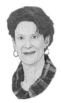 The avatar to the left represents Francine Campone, EdD. Francine shares her insights as a patient into the journey through two total hip replacements.

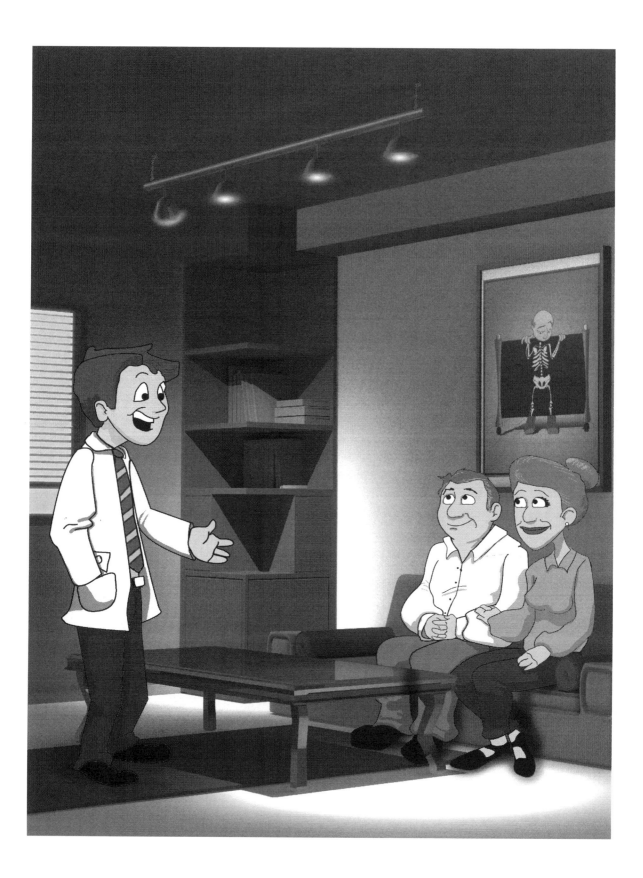

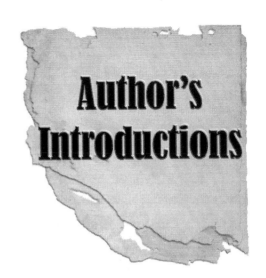

Dr. Hugate—

Welcome to *The Handbook of Hip and Knee Replacement!* It is my great pleasure to coauthor this handbook alongside one of my patients. This book is written as both a handbook and a guide through two very complex journeys that have a great deal in common: total hip replacement (THR) and total knee replacement (TKR). I think you'll find this handbook extremely informative and helpful in guiding you through the world of joint replacement surgery and in making important decisions regarding your function and quality of life.

In July 2009, I met a new patient in my office by the name of Robert Holland. Robert eventually underwent successful surgery on his painful knee. During routine follow-up exams, we took a few extra moments and discussed his struggles while researching basic information regarding joint replacement procedures. He explained to me that he was quite frustrated by the fact that it was so difficult to find good, reliable, and accurate information about the entire joint replacement process. He felt that much of the information available was either too technically oriented or written in such a way that the reader feels like a student being lectured by a professor and getting lost in the technical jargon.

I must admit, I was quite surprised. Up to that point, I had never tried to research joint replacements from a potential patient's perspective. I had no idea what information was out there for the general public's consumption. I suppose I just assumed that with the ease of access to information on the World Wide Web and thousands of medical blog sites, there would be an abundance of information. In fact there is, but it's a jumble to the ordinary layperson who is trying to gather both reliable and unbiased information and make sense of it. I was especially disturbed because, by this time, I realized through our various conversations that Robert was an extremely tech-savvy patient (as a technology professional throughout his career)—much more so than the average patient. I thought to myself, *if an information technology professional has a hard time finding information, it must be especially difficult for the average patient out there.*

I was living in my own world, reading technical journals and sharing ideas with colleagues regularly, but I was somewhat detached from what my patients were seeing, hearing, and finding with their own resources. It was this realization and subsequent discussions with Robert that led us to produce this handbook.

I have been an orthopedic surgeon for nine years and currently practice in Denver, Colorado. Every week I see patients in my clinic with painful hips and knees. I do my best to communicate all of the medical options and relevant points in an understandable way to my patients who are considering joint replacement surgery. Unfortunately, there are always some issues we're unable to clearly discuss and define during the brief visits in my office. This can be frustrating for both patient and physician, but is an unfortunate reality. This is why a "handbook" resource like this is invaluable. In our writing (and your reading) of this handbook, no longer is our discussion limited by time.

The Baby Boomers

The number of people worldwide considering joint replacement surgery is dramatically increasing. For the United States alone (based on the latest 2009 statistics from the Centers for Disease Control and Prevention [CDC]), for all patients and ages there will be more than 885,000 joint replacement procedures in the year 2012. This phenomenon has to do with several factors. In part, it's due to advances in medicine over the last few decades. Life expectancies continue to rise and are now well into the 70s in most developed countries; therefore, more people are "out-living their joints." In addition, enhanced expectations about the quality of life during the average person's retirement years continue to be higher as well. So, although people live longer, they also expect to *live better*—and that's where modern joint replacement procedures can help.

Another reason that we're seeing a vast increase in the number of joint replacements performed in the USA (and around the world) is that the so-called Baby Boomer generation is coming of age. These are the folks most likely to consider joint replacement. The most commonly accepted definition of the Baby Boomer generation is anybody born between the years 1946 and 1964. These are mostly children of military servicemen and women who decided to start a new family upon their return from overseas conflicts. As I write this book, this group of Americans ranges in age from about 47 to 65 years old.

If you are reading this handbook, you're most likely a member of the Baby Boomer generation and are probably considering the possibility of joint replacement surgery in the near or long term. If you're not a Baby Boomer yourself, then you probably have a family member or loved one who is considering joint replacement surgery, and we've also written this book with you in mind. Big decisions, such as the decision to undergo surgery, aren't made in a vacuum. The decision to have a joint replacement has to do with a number of factors and is fairly complex. It can (and does) also affect loved-ones in your life, as they're often called upon to help out physically and emotionally during recovery. Most of my patients depend on their immediate family and friends for advice and counsel regarding whether hip or knee replacement surgery is appropriate. Knowledge is power, and it is our hope that this book presents the complex subject of joint replacement in an understandable format with both the patient's and doctor's perspective, and allows people of all walks of life to make well-informed decisions about their medical treatment.

How this Handbook is Different

I think you'll find that this handbook is *different* from other information sources on joint replacement in a couple of very important ways. The first difference you'll notice while reading this book is that it's written by both patients *and* health care professionals. This is important, as most of the books available on this complex subject are typically written by one or the other. This handbook is also different in *how* it is written. It is written in plain language. We have not written this with a professorial tone, and we do not "talk down" to the reader like a parent to a child. We have made every attempt to use understandable language throughout. That is not to say that patients are incapable of understanding the issues. But when complex, technical, "medical jargon" is entered into the conversation, it can be hard for the layperson to follow. On the occasion that we need to use technical language to get our point across, we clearly explain what we mean by the phrases chosen. We have also included a glossary to help better define the vocabulary.

As you shall see, successful joint replacement surgery really is a *collaborative event* between patient and doctor, and I think the unique format of our book truly brings a fresh perspective to the process. There will be subjects in this book completely written by health professionals and others completely written by patients. We will insert comments from our different perspectives when appropriate to help you understand the entire subject more thoroughly. In short, we're interested in making a complex subject more approachable and understandable.

We were very fortunate to have Francine Campone, EdD, contribute her first-hand knowledge of two total hip replacements to our handbook. She and Robert (my co-author, who has undergone two knee replacements) bring to this manual very refreshing and practical patient's viewpoints, which you'll find very informative. I think you'll also find— if you choose to make this journey through total joint replacement—that what doctors think is important and what patients think is important *are not always the same*. This handbook does a good job of emphasizing both perspectives and therefore improving your understanding of the issues.

Being a doctor is a humbling experience—both a privilege and responsibility.

There is no greater honor than receiving the trust of a patient. Aside from the technical skills required to be a good doctor, we must remember to be good teachers. In fact the word "doctor" is the Latin word for "teacher". I hope to use this handbook to teach you about the issues surrounding hip and knee replacement and make the subject more understandable and accessible for you. In this handbook, we'll help you "cut through the fog," look through the hip and knee replacement journey from beginning to end, and try to bring you every pertinent point needed to make the important decisions along the way.

Thanks to you, the reader, for taking the time to participate in your care. As with most things in life, the more you put into it, the more you will get out of it.

Mr. Holland—

Greetings! We're excited you've chosen our handbook of hip and knee joint replacement because we feel very strongly that it will prepare you well should you decide to embark on this life-changing journey. Please allow me to introduce myself. I'm Robert Holland and I'm a certified Project Management Professional (PMP). I'm also an author of science fiction—one of my favorite avocations—and I have been a technical writer in the information technology industry for the last sixteen years of my professional life. I'm also the recipient of two knee replacements. It was my esteemed coauthor, Dr. Ronald R. Hugate Jr., who performed my knee replacement surgery in the middle of 2009.

Within the pages of this handbook, we've undertaken the daunting task of helping you gather the knowledge you need to understand the entire process of joint replacement. We want to share our wisdom to help you create a successful outcome for yourself, whether or not joint replacement surgery is the best path for you.

When my wife, Vicki, and I first met Dr. Hugate, I had been having chronic and quite bothersome troubles for several months from my first total knee replacement (TKR). My original orthopedic surgeon was baffled by my symptoms and referred us to Dr. Hugate, who is an expert in joint replacement surgery (among other things). He thoroughly examined me, and—after making his diagnosis—reviewed the options with us, explaining that the symptoms I was experiencing would quite likely improve with revision surgery on this knee. We also discussed options that did not require surgery. He explained to us that I could modify my life style by becoming less active and this would likely decrease my pain as well. As such, another surgery wasn't necessarily mandatory. He advised us of the potential benefits, explained the risks, and proffered his professional, medical opinion. We had many tough questions for him and he patiently and very thoroughly answered them.

The course you choose in finding and deciding what's best for you (and your family) while on your own life's journey should not be predetermined before you begin gathering your information. For this reason, I want to reinforce the idea of keeping an open mind:

Nowhere in this handbook do we assume that you will choose to embark on the journey through joint replacement. Rather, the theme of this handbook is to help you begin thinking clearly about your life, your loved ones, the options you have, what you want, where you wish to end up, and how best to get there.

Because Dr. Hugate didn't assume I would choose another joint replacement surgery and presented my choices as optional, our trust in him was greatly enhanced. He clearly wanted me to make the best decision for myself, and that was very important to us both as a couple. Vicki took very careful notes that day, and over the course of the following week, we considered the implications and examined our financial resources. We took into account my personal objectives and our desired life style (we love to hike and camp in the Colorado wilderness), and reviewed my current problems and limitations. Finally, after some lively discussion and careful deliberation, we decided that my best option was to proceed ahead with surgery.

The revision TKR went much better than the original. Dr. Hugate steered me skillfully through this second operation as surely as an experienced river rafting guide brings his boat full of innocent adventure seekers safely through the rapids. What a profound difference this was when compared to my first TKR experience! For example there is more than one way to manage post-operative pain and a number of options in anesthesia—none of which I knew before I had my second knee replacement and all of which are covered in this handbook. Throughout the next several months of routine checkups afterward (during which time I was thriving), we repeatedly discussed the idea that this whole journey could—and would—go a lot more smoothly if there was an easy-to-understand, yet comprehensive guidebook concerning joint replacement. This idea eventually took root and we decided to move forward in sharing our combined knowledge and wisdom.

In choosing us as your guides, you now have the keys to a comprehensive store of specific knowledge and wisdom about joint replacement.

By presenting and discussing all the salient points and sharing our knowledge and wisdom about these important matters, we've developed an up-to-date and very powerful handbook to guide and inform you as you work your own way through the decision-making process. Should you decide to proceed, our handbook is also written to help you prepare for and successfully navigate this profound course of events by knowing your options and cognitively choosing the best course forward—as opposed to floating down the river without a paddle (to rephrase and old saying). As you've no doubt noticed, I've been speaking about these often misunderstood and complex subjects like they're a raft trip down the river. So, let's explore and expand this idea some more, and have a little bit of fun as we do:

Going through joint replacement is a journey which starts and ends at home.

Life is a voyage on the big river. . . .

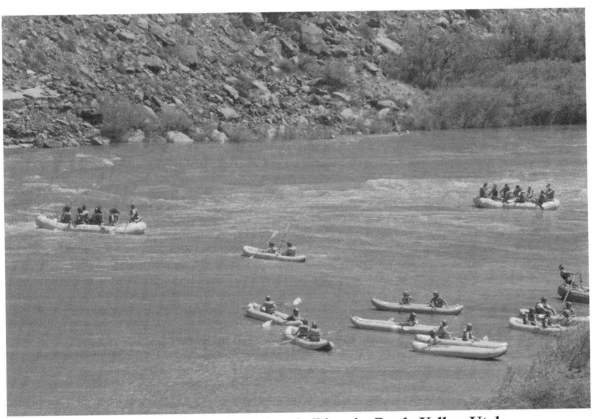

A rafting flotilla on the Colorado River in Castle Valley, Utah.

In the language of poetry, the previous two sentences are known as a metaphors and when combined, these two metaphors give us some nice tools for creating a friendly dialogue throughout our handbook by allowing us to refer to either hip replacement (THR) or knee replacement (TKR) as journeys.

So, let's begin now:

The choices you make while on your rafting trip down the river of life make all the difference in where you end up. Choosing to make the journey through joint replacement (or not) will make a profound difference in your life, and (either way) the outcome depends on you.

Of course, on any rafting trip there must be at least one person in the boat. Obviously this would be you if you're looking at THR or TKR, but chances are you're not the only one in the boat and, obviously, you're not alone on the river. While those closest and most important to you on this exceptional adventure are easily identified, there are others along the way who—while not so obvious—are nevertheless right there on the raft trip alongside you. It's easy to tell who these other *stakeholders* are by using the following definition (and we'll be using this term throughout our handbook):

Stakeholders on this journey are those who are committed to your well-being and success, those dependent upon you, or upon whom you depend, and, of course, those who love you and are helping you paddle the boat!

Assuming you are indeed committed to your own well-being, as the person considering this journey you would be the "primary stakeholder." The other stakeholders on this proposed journey are your spouse (life partner, or significant other), family, primary care provider (your family doctor), orthopedic surgeon (your specialist), nurses, physical and occupational therapists (and/or any other medical professionals involved in your care), and possibly others known only to you. Each has a role to play with a "positive interest" in the outcome. Each is fully prepared to help you define the questions, seek out the answers, review your decisions, and accompany, support, comfort, and encourage you, and sometimes even yell at you to paddle harder.

In planning to go on any rafting trip, there is always a comprehensive discussion concerning whether or not to start out in the first place, with the following question at the heart of it.

Can you handle the raft down this branch of the river?

We'll help you discover the answer to this important question and many others. So, before packing up your rucksack, canteen and grub, loading up the raft, jumping on and embarking on this new float trip, you will certainly have some important questions to answer and lots of planning to do and preparations to make as you work through your checklist. Simply put, just as anybody would evaluate their choices, plan, and prepare for such a floating trip, you must evaluate, plan and prepare for a joint replacement.

We're very lucky that we live in a time when a completely arthritic or worn out joint no longer means a life of sedentary decrepitude and weakness—lucky that we live in a time when we can even consider the choices described in this handbook. Therefore, I'll take a moment to speak about attitude and how it can affect your course. If you decide to embark on this journey, attitude makes the difference whether you're in a difficult and miserable experience paddling upstream or a bold and exciting adventure paddling easily along and happily going with the flow. Let's talk about the specific attitude that I know from experience will serve you best:

The outcome of your journey depends on your attitude as a proactive, determined, and committed patient.

A __proactive patient__ is one who actively participates throughout this journey and arms herself with all the knowledge she can obtain before starting out.

A __determined patient__ is one who has made up his mind to get the most out of this effort, and will not settle for half-hearted attempts or mediocre results.

A __committed patient__ is one who has decided to work carefully with— and listen carefully to—her surgeons, nurses, therapists, and health care providers, and do what's both needed and advised in the healthy spirit of cooperation.

If you adopt such a positive attitude as described above, the same attitude Dr. Hugate helped me find in my own time of need, you will journey well, knowing that the objective of your proactive determination and commitment is to enjoy an excellent float trip and nothing less! Now, let's look at the phases you will navigate in the joint replacement journey.

Planning (the key to success)

The importance of planning cannot be overstated because it guides and informs you throughout the upcoming stages of your journey. There's an old adage, "People don't plan to fail they fail to plan." Planning is a time of knowledge gathering, of putting aside fears and anxiety in favor of healthy curiosity, of comprehensively identifying all of your stakeholders. Use their knowledge and wisdom to help you decide whether or not to proceed. If, during this period of knowledge gathering and counsel, you decide to proceed, you'll begin even more extensive planning.

This is the period of time when all of the very important questions are asked and fully answered. Important people in your life are considered and educated alongside of you as important stakeholders in the outcome. Those who can help you find answers are consulted and their counsel given appropriate thought. Finally, the course forward is the result of comprehensive knowledge gathering so you may embark on your journey with confidence and a positive attitude.

Preparation (the other key to success)

If, after getting your questions answered, consulting with all the stakeholders, and resolving your concerns by completing the initial planning, you have decided to move forward, it's time to prepare for success.

Preparing for a successful joint replacement is complicated and involves a determined commitment to understanding and preparing for all practical, medical, and financial aspects. If you've read (and made sure you understand) all of the matters we've laid out in this handbook, you'll be very well informed and ready to embark on this life enhancing journey.

Joint Replacement (the commitment is made)

After all of your planning and preparations are completed and your home is readied, the day of surgery has come.

You check into the hospital well prepared, knowing what to expect and feeling comfortable with all of your choices. Your chosen surgeon and his team perform the operation, the wonderful hospital treatment team takes great care of you, and before long, you're checking out and going home.

After Joint Replacement (a life reclaimed)

Coming home from the hospital signals the beginning of the serious work involved with recovering, but also the joyful work of getting on with the rest of your life. In the short term (for the next month or two), you have a great deal of hard work ahead of you. In the long term, you will develop new routines and habits based on the type of replacement you have. As you learn once more to enjoy your life based on the renewed strength you've painstakingly built, you begin to explore and enjoy your life's journey, which is no longer dominated by a painful hip or knee joint.

Every day after surgery is the first day of the rest of your life. At first, it's about the hard work of getting back to normal, regaining your strength once again, reclaiming your happiness, and forgetting about all the pain and problems associated with that painful worn out old joint. As time goes by, you realize that you have created a bright new future and are working happily to build new prosperity and find new joys.

To sum up, this journey began as pain—subtle at first—maybe as a twinge after the morning tennis match, or an ache after the evening walk. You may have suffered an injury, or a series of surgical events on an already painful joint. This discomfort grew slowly and inexorably worse. By the time I came to my own decision to embark on this journey, every single step I took was a brutally painful reminder of what I was slowly losing.

10

As I went through my own journey, I would have given anything for a handbook such as this.

The authors and collaborators of this handbook all hope you find this material illuminating and empowering as we shed some light on the people, processes, and journey. We'll prepare you as best we can and (hopefully) give you enough information to make the best decision for you and the people you love.

We wish you all the best!

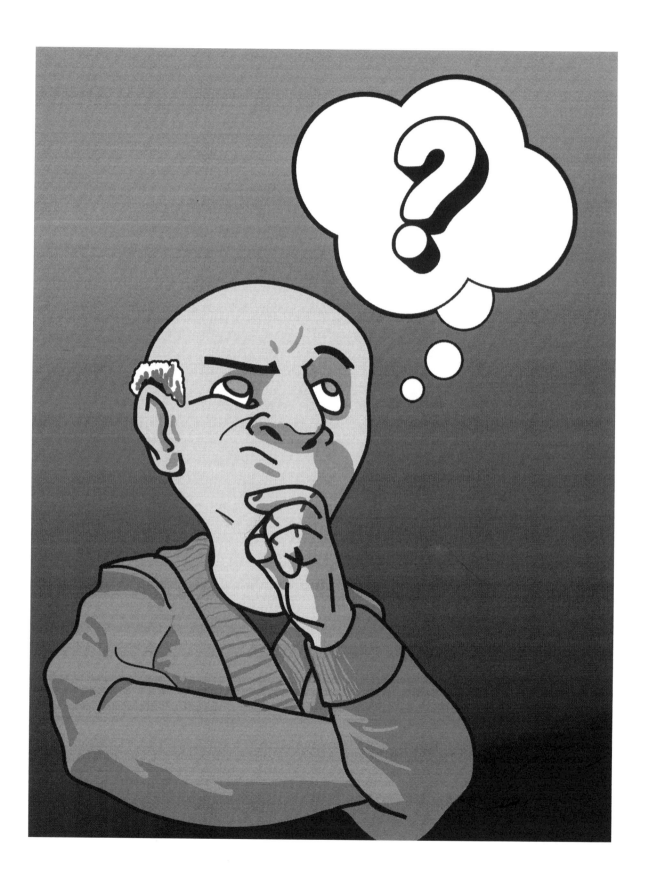

When Do You "Need" a Joint Replacement?

CHAPTER

1

by Dr. Hugate and Mr. Holland

Dr. Hugate—

On a clear Denver morning in mid-September, I met a nice couple who had driven up from Parker, Colorado, for an office visit. She was a proud grandmother, with two wonderful daughters who were both nurses. He was her devoted husband of over forty years. One of their daughters lived and worked in the Denver area and drove the two of them to her appointment. They didn't like doctor's visits, and they certainly didn't like city driving. The two of them lived in Georgia, but spent their summers in Colorado to be near their daughter (and grandchildren) and to get away from the heat and humidity of the southeast United States during the summer. They both spoke with a deep southern drawl. Fortunately, being from Virginia myself, I was able to translate and understand every word they said! I even brought back a bit of my own Southern accent to make them feel more at home. They had worked hard all of their lives and were planning to enjoy retirement watching their children and grandchildren grow.

"Doc, she's just not the same since her knees went bad," he said. I could tell he was worried about his bride of 40 years. It became clear to me that she had been encouraged to come to my office by their daughter, who was concerned.

"What exactly do you mean?" I asked.

"Well, she doesn't even like to go shopping anymore," he said. "She can hardly go for a simple walk. She's seems depressed, doesn't really want to go out and do anything because of the pain. Do you think she needs a knee replacement?"

This conversation, or some close variant, occurs regularly at my clinic and at clinics across around the world every day. It involves people at the end of their rope—no longer enjoying life because of the pain in their joints. This patient went on to have her knees replaced and has a new lease on life. She's one of my favorite patients because of her love for life, wonderful supportive family, and unmistakable southern drawl. The choice to have her knees replaced was the right one for her.

This chapter of our handbook deals with the million-dollar question:

When do you "need" to have a joint replacement?

This question is somewhat misleading, and you will see why after we discuss a few issues. We'll go over the various symptoms that patients with arthritis may experience and the differing forms of treatment. There are a number of less invasive treatments that should be considered before opting for hip or knee replacement and we'll review some of those as well.

Categories of Surgery

Let's start the discussion with some background. In general, there are two categories of surgery that we surgeons perform. The first is called *non-elective* surgery. This is a surgical procedure performed that is usually urgently necessary. Now you may stop and think to yourself, "Isn't all surgery necessary?" or "Why would you have surgery that is not necessary?" and these are both reasonable questions, but there are some surgeries that *must* be done and some that do not *need* to be performed. Let's look at an example.

Suppose one night I am on trauma call at my hospital and a patient comes in who was involved in a car accident and suffered a broken thighbone. That person needs an urgent, non-elective surgery to fix the bone. This is to say: The patient has no reasonable alternative to having surgery, and refusing to have surgery will certainly result in a worsening condition. They are not deciding of their independent will to have the surgery. The condition and subsequent surgery are thrust upon them because of the car accident. Unfortunately, there is no great alternative to having surgery in this example. There isn't much time for the patient to think about the decision, nor is there time for the patient to meet and discuss the issues with the doctor. There is virtually no opportunity for them to build mutual trust. This is the general nature of non-elective surgery. Clearly, it is not an ideal situation.

In contrast, *elective* surgery is a much more controlled situation. Fortunately, the vast majority of surgeries performed in the USA are elective. These are surgeries which are done under non-urgent, non-emergency conditions. The patient and doctor are under no time constraints, so they have time to meet, consider the patient's condition, gather information, and make a decision about surgery. There is opportunity for a second and perhaps third opinion if necessary. This is a much more desirable set of circumstances for both patient and doctor. It allows us, as physicians, enough time to make an accurate diagnosis and present all options so that the patient can make an informed decision with which she is comfortable. It allows time for the doctor and patient to develop a gut feeling for each other and creates the foundation for a trusting relationship.

One extreme example of an elective surgery is cosmetic surgery. If a person doesn't like the shape of his nose or the wrinkles on his face, he has the option of consulting a plastic surgeon and considering elective plastic surgery. The condition he has is not dangerous or life-threatening. There is no urgency. The patient can read about the procedure and get one or multiple opinions from his plastic surgeons of choice. During visits with his surgeons, the patient can gather information on the alternatives and risks of surgery. Other issues such as healing time, back-to-work time, and the amount of pain can be discussed. Once the patient feels he has enough information about the advantages and disadvantages of having the surgery, he can elect to have the surgery or not. You would (or should) never be told that you "need" to have a nose job or a face-lift. The decision to have this type of surgery is based on your perceived quality of life and whether going through the risk and pain of surgery outweighs remaining in your current condition.

Now let's discuss arthritis and joint replacement. Joint replacement is considered an elective procedure for those suffering from severe arthritis that is not responsive to medical treatment. What is arthritis? Well, *arthritis* literally means "inflammation of the joint." Inflammation is the body's natural response to injury. The classic inflammatory signs and symptoms of arthritis include pain, warmth, swelling, and sometimes redness. Osteoarthritis is the most common form of arthritis, but there are others. *Osteoarthritis* refers specifically to that type of arthritis that is present in "worn out" joints. In this sense of our definition, the cartilage—essentially the cushion between the bones—is generally severely worn and may even be gone, which results in bare-bone rubbing on bare-bone. From this point on, throughout our handbook, when we say "arthritis," we will assume we are talking about "osteoarthritis."

The fluid in the knee (called synovial fluid) is more watery in those with arthritis and no longer provides adequate lubrication. The bone may even form "spurs" in response to the presence of the arthritis. People with arthritic joints typically develop worsening joint pain over the course of many years. In those with knee arthritis, the pain is generally centered in the knee. For those with hip arthritis the pain is usually felt in the groin. This is not a dangerous or life-threatening condition, but it does HURT. Some people also develop deformities such as "bowed-legs" or "knock-knees" that worsen over years as well. People with arthritis may also develop "fluid on the knee" (sometimes also known as "water on the knee") especially after they are active.

As I mentioned, there are other forms of arthritis. *Rheumatoid arthritis*, for example, can be extremely debilitating. This is a type of arthritis called "auto-immune." In basic terms, this means that the body's immune system sees its own normal cartilage as a foreign invader—and mounts an attack. This destroys the cartilage and leads to pain and deformity. Patients with rheumatoid arthritis can eventually come to need a joint replacement, but their treatment regimens are much more complex than that of patients with osteo-arthritis. Any patient with rheumatoid arthritis should be under the watchful care of a rheumatologist, a physician who specializes in the diagnosis and medical treatment of auto-immune diseases. The rheumatologist knows when or if all medical options have been exhausted and will make a referral to a joint replacement surgeon when appropriate.

Regardless of the type, the pain from arthritis progressively worsens to the point where people with this severe condition just give up the things they enjoy doing. Going for walks with their spouse (or significant other), playing with grandkids, or simply going shopping all become too painful. As a result, people can become depressed and frustrated by the condition. If you feel this describes your current symptoms and outlook on life, the first step is to see your primary care provider (PCP) for examination to confirm the diagnosis of arthritis.

Options for Treatment of Arthritis

Do Nothing

What are your options if you have arthritis? The first option is no treatment at all. This is the option with the least risk, but it does not address the pain. Again, arthritis is not dangerous or life-threatening, so for patients who are willing (and able) to tolerate the pain, and do not want to try medications or injections, this is an option. If you have taken the time to go to the doctor's office for treatment, however, you have probably already crossed the threshold for seeking relief.

Activity Modification and Weight Loss

The next option is that of activity modification and weight loss. This essentially means you must stop doing what hurts and lose weight—easier said than done. The nature of arthritis is that it is more painful when you are more active.

So, not surprisingly, people with painful joints are less likely to exercise, and therefore more likely to gain weight. This weight gain makes their pain worse and they decrease activities even more. This lack of activity (and subsequent psychological depression in some cases) may cause even more weight gain and make the pain even worse, and so on. It can turn into a vicious cycle. People I see who are morbidly obese (the most extreme medical category of obesity), I counsel on weight loss and even, on occasion, send them to see a weight-loss specialist to consider gastric banding or gastric bypass (so-called stomach stapling) to help them lose the weight. This may seem like a radical approach, but being extremely obese can significantly increase your risk for medical or surgical complications.

Physical Therapy

Physical therapy can be helpful in the early stages of arthritis in that it can strengthen and increase the flexibility of the hip or knee. Physical therapists can also help with weight loss strategies through the use of off-loaded exercises. For example, water-therapy is physical therapy in a pool, which can give you a good aerobic workout without irritating your joints.

Medication

The next step in treatment generally involves the use of medications. Medications that can be effective against arthritic pain include acetaminophen (Tylenol); nonsteroidal anti-inflammatory drugs (aka NSAIDS), such as ibuprofen (Advil), naproxen (Aleve), ketoprofen (Orudis), and celecoxib (Celebrex); and mild narcotic pain medications, such as Vicodin or codeine. In general, especially in the earlier stages of arthritis, pain is intermittent or occurs in "flare-ups". If this is the case, then managing these flare-ups using medications alone often proves sufficient. For example, if you have arthritic knee pain and are planning to go on a hike that you know will aggravate your knee, it's a good idea to pre-medicate yourself with Tylenol or your NSAID of choice beforehand and for a short period after the activity.

The problem is that as arthritic pain progresses, it is generally more severe and long-standing—which requires more medication for a longer time. And although these medications are generally not dangerous when used short-term, they all become more dangerous with long-term use in ever-increasing doses. All medications have potential side effects. Acetaminophen, for example, can cause liver problems among other things with prolonged use. Anti-inflammatories can cause stomach irritation, or even stomach ulcers. On rare occasion anti-inflammatories can cause kidney or liver problems. Narcotic pain medications like codeine are all derivatives of morphine or heroin (known as opiates) and can work well in the short term, but can be addictive when used longer term. Because of the effects that narcotics may have on your brain, you may experience slowed or delayed thought while on them as well. Unfortunately, none of these medications addresses or removes the cause of the pain. They simply mask or reduce the symptoms. For that reason, medications may not be a good long-term solution in patients with severe arthritis.

Joint Injections

The next more aggressive treatment option is that of injecting medications into the joint. This is the first of the "invasive options" for arthritis treatment. That is, the first option that requires a break in the skin- in this case with a needle. While this is a reasonable option in those with knee arthritis, it is less so in those with hip arthritis. The knee is a joint that is easily and safely accessible by injection because of its location. The hip is harder to inject (because it is a deeper joint) and is more painful and difficult to inject because there are some important nerves and blood vessels near the hip joint. For that reason, while we *can* inject the hip, it is generally less desirable to perform injections in the hip joint.

There are several different types of injections but they fall into two overall categories. In general, there are those that contain steroids, and those that are lubricants (so-called viscosupplementation). Steroid injections are often mixed with numbing medications and injected directly into the joint to provide a strong anti-inflammatory effect. The steroids used are not muscle-building steroids, but are a steroid family called *corticosteroids*. These are potent, anti-inflammatory substances that can be effective especially when injected directly at the site of the inflammation (inside the arthritic joint). There are dozens of steroids that can be used and it usually boils down to the doctor's preference as to which one you'll get. Steroids often take a few days to start working and some steroids can even make the pain worse for a day or two before taking effect.

In general, the effect of the steroid is proportional to the severity of arthritis. If you have severe arthritis, the shots may last only for a week or two. In milder arthritis, the shots may provide relief for months. I have patients who do very well with injections over the short term. For example, they may come in to get a shot before a vacation (or other life event) to help them get through it without pain. Over the long term, though, as the arthritis worsens, shots tend to give less pain relief and for a shorter time. We tend to limit the number of injections of steroids over time because the steroids can weaken ligaments and tendons if given too frequently. For that reason, I limit my patients to two injections per year. Injections into the joints generally do not get into the blood stream in large amounts and therefore these are safe for diabetics, although those patients may see a very slight increase in blood sugars for a day or two after the injection.

The other common type of injection is *viscosupplementation*. Think of these injections as lubrication for the joint—like motor oil for the car. The joint fluid in arthritis patients is generally more "watery" and less viscous than normal joint fluid and does not lubricate the joint well. The injected fluid is quite viscous (like heavy oil or honey) and is placed directly into the joint to temporarily replace or supplement the joint fluid. These shots improve the viscosity and relieve pain in this manner. The main ingredient in most of these is *hyaluronic acid*, which is a substance normally found in the joint. Some of these are one-time injections and some require a series of three to five weekly injections. Again, similar to steroid injections, the effect is temporary and dependent on the severity of the arthritis. I generally offer these injections when patients have at least some cartilage remaining. Once the cartilage is worn out completely, it has been my experience that viscous supplementation does not work well. There have also been rare instances of allergic reactions to the shots which can actually worsen the pain and inflammation. This usually occurs during the second or subsequent injections after the first series of shots have been given. Because the hyaluronic acid is manufactured from rooster combs (yes, you read that correctly), you should let your doctor know prior to getting any injections if you're allergic to chickens, eggs, or products containing these ingredients.

Joint Replacement

If you have tried these lesser-invasive options, and none of them worked well enough for you—and you are in reasonable health—then you are considered a candidate for joint replacement. Remember, per our prior discussion, this is an elective procedure. We will focus on the surgeries themselves later in the manual but for now let's address the title of this chapter... the million dollar question:

Do I need a joint replacement?

The answer I always give is:

Only you can tell me that.

It may seem like I'm dodging the question, but it is absolutely true! Aside from some extreme examples, it is rare that you would ever *need* to have a joint replacement for medical reasons. It usually boils down to this:

Is your current quality of life acceptable to you? Does the amount of pain and limited function you are experiencing warrant going through surgery and recovery with the risks associated?

Here are a couple of questions you should ask yourself—that my patients find helpful when deciding whether to have surgery:

Do I wake up in the morning and have to plan my day around my hip or knee? Are there things that I enjoy doing that I don't do today because my hips (or knees) hurt too badly?

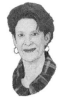 **Campone's Comment:** It may even be useful to consider another question before Dr. Hugate's first, "Did discomfort in my joint interfere with me getting a good night's sleep?" As I discuss later, sleep is a critical component of a good quality of life and lack of sleep has a negative domino effect on all aspects of your waking life. ~*~

If the answer to any of these questions is yes, then you should, in my opinion, consider joint replacement surgery. Of course, surgery will not make your joint normal again, but it generally does a great job of relieving pain and improving the quality of your life. We will discuss these issues in detail later in this handbook, and cover the benefits and risks of joint replacement surgery, and what limitations you will have after joint replacement.

20

This, along with my descriptions of the procedures and anticipated recoveries should give you enough information so that you can weigh whether joint replacement is the right thing for you. This is an elective procedure, so take all the time you need to make the right decision. Include your medical caregivers, family members, and trusted friends in your decision as well.

Remember, there are other causes for pain in your joints. It's also important to realize that the discussion we're having here pertains only to those with severe osteoarthritis of the hip or knee. There are certainly causes for hip and knee pain other than osteoarthritis, and these may require different treatments. Gout, pinched nerves, rheumatoid arthritis, avascular necrosis (AVN), and cartilage tears are examples of other common causes of joint pain—just to name a few. It's important that you have a physician assess your painful joint, using your medical history, physical examinations, X-rays, and various laboratory tests (as needed) to ensure that osteoarthritis is indeed the cause of your pain so you can receive the correct diagnosis and advice for a course of treatment.

Mr. Holland—

My story starts many years before I actually knew I'd be writing this handbook. As a construction man in the various trades, I spent most of my life going up and down ladders. I once calculated that I made the round trip on an eight-foot (or higher) ladder, wearing a heavy tool belt, over 100,000 times throughout the early years of my life. Will this wear out your knees? You bet it will! Then, in the late 1980s, I had an opportunity to return to college, and by the time I graduated, I was in my mid-40s. It was the beginning of the end for my knee because the damage was already done. However, being a tough-guy ex-sailor from the Vietnam Era and a former construction man, I limped onward through my life, tolerating the slowly yet ever-increasing pain. At times it even became difficult to do something as simple as going for a walk at the mall.

In the late 1990s, my knee pain became so bad that I had a surgery performed in which the torn cartilage was trimmed, and free-floating cartilage debris inside the knee joint was removed. This procedure is known as *Arthroscopy*. After that, things improved temporarily for the next eight to nine years, and then began getting more and more painful. By late 2008 when I was in my late 50s, I was experiencing severe pain from virtually all of the things I love to do, such as bicycling, hiking, working out in the gym, and going for a mall-crawl in the winter—even shopping for groceries. I was to the point that I couldn't get down out of my pickup truck with the bad knee first, and I couldn't climb into my pickup using the bad knee. Further, I was in agony going up and coming down the stairs in my own house.

There were other compelling issues which, for me, created the tipping point and drove my decision to have my knee joint replaced. Anybody who owns their own home knows there are day-to-day maintenance issues which can easily be done by the homeowner or can be quite expensive when hired out. I got to a point where whenever I went up the ladder to my roof, I had to go one leg at a time, with my good knee always carrying the work-load. Getting back on that ladder afterward was dicey as well. This became an obvious safety issue. While on the roof I had trouble keeping my footing and staying upright. Further, I found I was unable to mow the lawn anymore. Honestly, I could make a long list of these types of activities around the house, but there's no need—you get the picture.

Then, there eventually came the most heartbreaking loss of quality in my life. You see, I am an outdoorsman, I've had a deep love of the outdoors all of my life. That's one of the reasons I live in Colorado. Thus, as the osteoarthritis in my knee progressed, by the time I was 58 years old, I came to a point where I could no longer enjoy an ordinary, moderate hike in the mountains near Denver. My knee would ache fiercely all night long after a hike and, for me, this was the last straw.

Hugate's Comment: An important point to make here is how your age may factor into decisions regarding your hip or knee treatment. At the point where Robert's knee began hurting him (in his thirties and forties), he would have been too young to consider a joint replacement. As I write this handbook, joint replacements last about fifteen years on average. For that reason, we tend to discourage people younger than fifty years old from getting their joints replaced. Why? Younger people are more active and tend to wear their joint replacements out faster. When the joint replacement is worn out, you may need to have surgery to fix or replace the worn piece(s), which is called revision joint replacement surgery. This can add up to multiple revision surgeries if you get your first joint replacement in your forties. If you have knee pain like this at a young age, the treatments of choice are non-surgical, as outlined in my portion of this chapter.

Robert also gives an excellent description here of the progressively worsening nature of severe arthritis and how it became unbearable in his late fifties. His words are those of a man at the end of his rope. Simple things became difficult. An otherwise healthy man, full of life, found it difficult to walk in a mall. Given his described level of function and pain, Robert was right to consider knee replacement surgery at this point in his life. ~*~

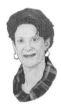

Campone's Comment: This progression is not unique to knees. In **Chapter 6, Journey through Two Hip Replacements,** I observe that there's a slow, but noticeable decline in the ability to comfortably go about ordinary, functional activities and increasing interference with critical functions like the ability to sleep.

One aspect of the process to be aware of is known as "boiled frog syndrome." Because of the gradual erosion of mobility and ease in day-to-day activities, it's possible to overlook the increasing erosion of quality of life and changes in personality resulting from the stress of constantly managing the discomfort. The analogy comes from the widespread anecdote that if you drop a frog into boiling water, it will immediately jump out. However, If you put it in a pot of cool water and gradually raise the temperature degree-by-degree, the frog gets used to the change and gets cooked. As Robert and Dr. Hugate both note, family members are sometimes the first ones to notice and point out the need for action.

In considering the decision about readiness, individuals might want to consider two aspects of the joint pain in their day-to-day experience: pervasiveness and permanence. Pervasiveness means how many different life activities are affected by the pain and limited mobility. In my case, I didn't mind having to sit out on dancing and exercise classes. However, when all forms of movement were not just uncomfortable but painful, things reached a tipping point. Similarly, permanence of the discomfort is a factor. When pain can be alleviated by some of the non-surgical means that Dr. Hugate discusses, the condition is unpleasant but intermittent. When noticeable pain is a constant factor, there is often a psychological toll. Again, in my case, I noticed (and my nearest friends and colleagues did as well), an increased irritability, shortness of temper, impatience and a general sense of depression. It was this impact as much as my own physical experience that prompted me to say yes to the surgery. ~*~

However, this was not the only developing problem, as you will see. My other, relatively good knee was carrying almost the entire load. Even though it had never been operated on—and was in relatively good condition for my age—I was beginning to feel the wear and tear of using the good knee to compensate for the bad. Moreover, other parts of my body were also casualties of my bad knee. My hip and buttocks on the right side were very weak and undeveloped. These muscles were withering away. This was surprising to me because I'm a really active person. This meant that my pelvis had tilted from so many years of limping and that tilt threw my entire back out of alignment as well. Therefore, along with my knee pain, my entire back was a train wreck and I was deep in the well of constant pain. In fact, I'd been this way for so long, I didn't even know I was limping all the time.

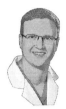

Hugate's Comment: This is a common issue seen in those with severe arthritis of the hip or knee. Pain causes you to alter your gait, and this alteration in your gait causes new stresses on your "good" joints. Pretty soon you may have pain in your good knee or back pain as a result. It is a cycle of pain commonly seen in those with end-stage arthritis of their joints. ~*~

Finally, I went to my local orthopedic surgeon to see if I could get some relief. When I got there, he did a full examination of my knees and informed me I had end-stage osteoarthritis. Dr. Hugate explained the condition, but I want to describe just how severely this can hurt! I'm talking about some very, very bright pain in my leg and back, severe grinding in the knee so bad it seemed to make my teeth chatter, and heavy pain in my back so severe I was barely able to cope with my day-to-day life. The surgeon told me I needed to consider a total knee replacement and "get that bad knee joint out of there." This was not what I wanted to hear. Obviously, it was time to start doing some research. I only wish I could have read a great handbook like this back then.

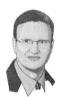

Hugate's Comment: Remember that joint replacement is an elective procedure and rarely urgent. Robert did the right thing here by taking a deep breath, stepping back, and discover-ing his options. ~*~

Before my own journey through TKR, I spent a great deal of time on the World Wide Web studying the various implants, issues, and possibilities. There are the typical manufacturer's claims about longevity of their implant and superiority of their installa-tion methodology and so on. Much of this was subjective (versus objective) information. What's more, if you do some Internet research for yourself, you'll also notice that each of these websites provides lots of generic information about the processes of aging and arthritis while subtlety mixing in how their implant is the best fix. It makes sense for them to promote their products—but realize it's their sales pitch. It's up to you to wade through the information and do your best to figure out what's good science versus good marketing.

So let's examine my desired outcome—and we'll assume it is yours as well. Simply put, what I wanted was to get a new lease on life and return to greater health through the freedom of long-term, improved mobility and the absence of constant, debilitating pain. I wanted to discover the enhancement of my lifestyle by regaining what age, work, accidents, and health problems took away. I still think of these stated objectives as my "mission statement" throughout my own journey through TKR—which is a rafting trip I am now enjoying to the fullest.

In making your decision, spend some time understanding your current limitations and where they come from. Think very carefully about what you're willing to accept in terms of desired activities versus limited behavior (based on intolerable pain levels). Then, strike a balance between knowing when you're in enough pain that it's downgrading your life in unacceptable ways and sensing when it's time to take corrective action. In my case, the decision was crystal clear but a long time in the making, and I spent some serious time studying everything I could without the benefit of a handbook such as this.

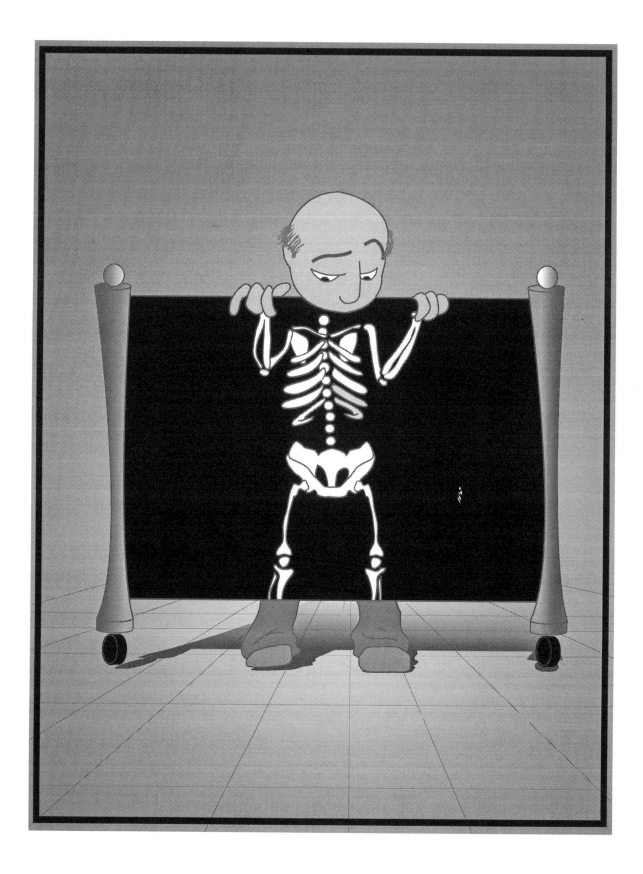

Nuts and Bolts of the Hip & Knee

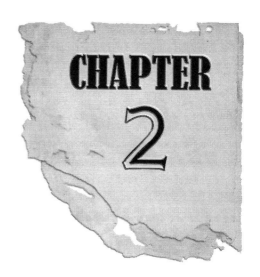

CHAPTER 2

by Dr. Hugate

Orthopedic surgeons go through years of training to learn the detailed and complex anatomy of the various joints of the body. I promise that I will *not* put you through that. I do think that if you're considering hip or knee replacement, you'll want to at least have an idea of what it is we are replacing. Don't worry, there will be no quiz at the end and I won't go into extreme detail—but we should talk about the "nuts and bolts" of the hip and knee joints. Some of this you will know and some will be new to you. In addition to describing the joint, we'll also include diagrams and X-rays to better illustrate things. I am a firm believer that "a picture is worth a thousand words." Being able to visualize your joints may give you more insight into what's gone wrong and how a joint replacement may help.

Basic Terminology

To help you understand some of the language your surgeon may use, let's go over the basic terms of anatomy and physiology. You will see these terms often when body parts and function are described throughout our handbook. You'll find all of these terms in the glossary of this handbook, but it's useful to discuss them here and help you into the right mindset.

We describe the study of the human body using two basic categories:

> ***Anatomy*** *is the science of describing the parts of the body.*
>
> ***Physiology*** *is the science of describing how those parts work.*

We describe the position of a specific structure in anatomy with the following terms:

Medial refers to any body part that is closer to the midline of your body.

Lateral refers to something that is further away from the midline of your body.

Anterior refers to a body part toward the front of your body.

Posterior refers to something that is toward the back of your body.

We describe motion of joints using the following terms:

Flexion refers to how a joint bends.

Extension refers to how a joint straightens out.

Because the knee has predominantly one plane of motion (like a hinge joint) we can use flexion and extension to describe the motion of the knee. The hip joint, being a ball-and-socket joint, is also capable of rotation, and we'll therefore use that descriptor as well. In terms of "stability," when a joint is solid and doesn't "give out," it is said to be a *stable* joint. On the other hand, if your joint feels "wobbly" or "gives out" on you, this may be because it's loose or *unstable*.

For clarity, let's define what joints are. Joints occur wherever bones come together in the body. The function of a joint is to connect bones. Most joints allow for some degree of motion. They usually connect two bones but there are a few joints that connect multiple bones, like the wrist joint. The type and degree of motion in joints will vary. For example, there are joints in the pelvis which move very little (like the sacroiliac joints), while other joints can move quite a bit, like a universal joint in all directions (for example the shoulder joint). Some act as a ball-and-socket (like the hip joint) and some act more like a hinge (the knee joint). Highly mobile joints like the knee and hip are called synovial joints. Synovial joints have thick capsules that surround them and contain the lubricating fluid within the joint, like motor oil for your car engine.

The basic elements of any synovial joint include the following:

Articular cartilage: the slick, rubbery coating on the end of a bone that helps cushion the point where the bones come together.

Tendons: strong bands of tissue that connect muscles to bones.

Ligaments: *strong bands of tissue that connect bones to other bones.*

Synovial fluid: *a slippery, viscous fluid within any synovial joint that helps provide lubrication.*

Joint capsule: *a thick wall of flexible tissue that surrounds a joint, helps stabilize it, and keeps the synovial fluid within it.*

When we reach early adulthood, the average thickness of our articular cartilage is about 4 mm. This cartilage is full of proteins and water and makes an extremely effective lubricated cushion for the knee joint. Synovial joints (like the hip and knee) are among the most well lubricated surfaces in the natural world. In fact, the cartilage and fluid in a normal knee are ten times slipperier than ice, or even Teflon. Amazing!

Knee Joint Anatomy

The knee is an example of a joint that roughly works like a hinge (though in reality the motion at the knee joint is more complex than a simple hinge). In the case of the knee, the hinge connects the *tibia* (leg bone) to the *femur* (thigh bone).

The X-ray below shows how these bones fit together (**See Figure 2.1**). The usual range of the motion of the knee is from full extension (straightening of the knee) at 0 degrees to about 130 degrees of flexion (bending of the knee).

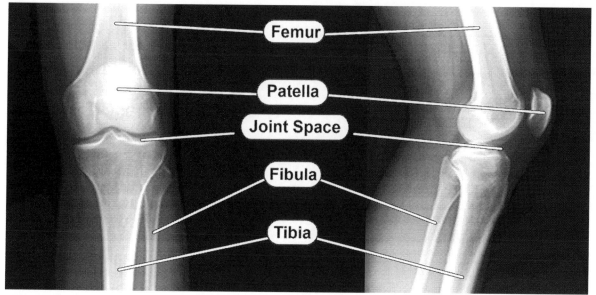

Figure 2.1 X-ray of the knee joint, front and side views

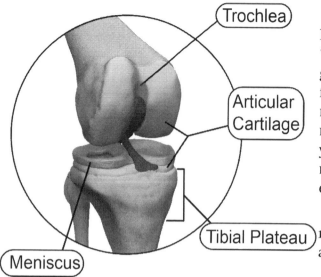

Figure 2.2 Anatomy of the knee

Many people can extend their knee slightly beyond straight (known as 'hyperextension') but the knee, in general, should not hyperextend very far. There is also a small amount of rotation that occurs at the knee as it moves. This occurs mostly whenever you engage in any type of pivoting motion. However, most people don't even know this is happening.

The top of the tibial surface is relatively flat and therefore is referred to as the *tibial plateau* (**See Figure 2.2**).

The end of the femur is shaped almost like a sweeping "W," with two rounded protrusions again called condyles. The one on the inside of the knee is referred to as the *medial condyle* and the one on the outer part of the knee is the *lateral condyle*.

The other bone that comprises the knee joint is the *patella* (commonly called the "kneecap"). It too has cartilage on the undersurface (aka *posterior surface*), and it is often the victim of arthritis and the culprit of pain in the front of the knee (**See Figure 2.3**). The patella sits in a groove on the front of the femur called the *trochlea* (**See Figure 2.2**). The trochlea guides the position of the patella through the full-range motion of the knee.

The bones of the knee joint are all coated with articular cartilage, as we discussed above. In the knee, however, there is an additional set of cartilages (**See Figure 2.2**) interposed between the femur and the tibia called the *meniscus* (or the plural form: *menisci*). The menisci are made of a different type of cartilage, but this cartilage serves

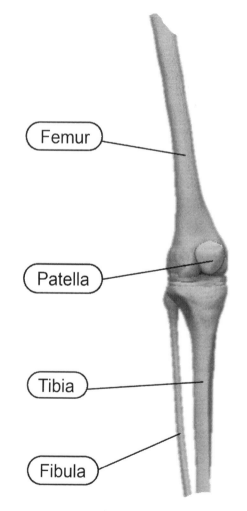

Figure 2.3 Bones of the lower extremity

a similar purpose. The menisci each have a "C" shape and act as a cradle to help create a better fit between the surfaces of the tibia and femur. If not for the menisci, the rounded femoral condyles would sit on the relatively flat tibial plateau and this would create a single point of contact and high stress that would quickly lead to joint breakdown and failure. Orthopedic surgeons prior to the 1980s would routinely take out the entire meniscus if it was injured (due to a lack of understanding at that time of how important the meniscus was to the knee joint). A lot of those patients are getting knee replacements today.

What holds the knee joint together? There are a few things that keep the knee stable and prevent it from being "wobbly." The most important stabilizers of the knee are the *ligaments*. Think of ligaments like strong, thick rubber bands that connect one bone to another. There are several in the knee (**See Figure 2.4**), and each has its own important function. The knee joint is stabilized from side-to-side motion by the *collateral ligaments*. These ligaments connect across the inner and outer aspects of the knee. The one on the inside of the knee is the *medial collateral ligament* (MCL) and the one on the outer part of the knee is called the *lateral collateral ligament* (LCL). There are also two important ligaments that cross in the center of the knee. Because they cross, they are called the *cruciate* ligaments. The one in the front is called the *anterior cruciate ligament* (ACL) and the one in the back is called the *posterior cruciate ligament* (PCL). The cruciate ligaments are important for stabilizing the knee in the front-to-back direction. They also primarily stabilize the knee against twisting action. Injury of any of these ligaments (to include stretching or tearing) can cause the knee to be unstable.

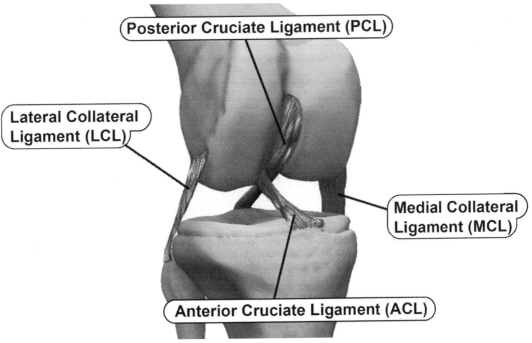

Figure 2.4 Ligaments of the knee

We surgeons think of the knee joint as having three separate *compartments* (**See Figure 2.5**). The first is the *medial compartment*. This is the space between the medial condyle of the femur and the medial tibial plateau. This is the part of the joint most commonly involved in osteoarthritis. The second is the *lateral compartment*, which is the space between the lateral femoral condyle and the lateral tibial plateau. The third compartment is the space between the patella and the femur; we call this the *patello-femoral compartment*. In most cases of advanced arthritis, all three compartments will show thinning of cartilage and signs of degradation and pain.

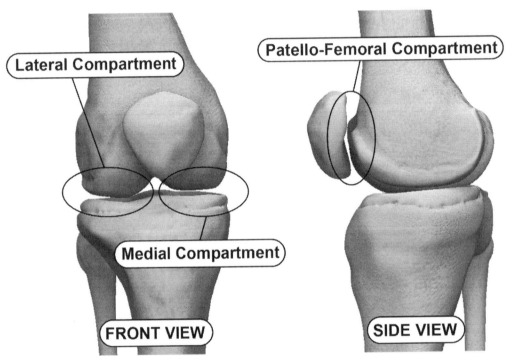

Figure 2.5 Compartments of the knee

There are rare occasions in which only one of the three compartments may have arthritis, and for those situations there are different knee replacement designs that replace only the affected part of the knee (so-called "partial" knee replacement). We will discuss this further in **Chapter 12, Methods, Types & Designs of Joint Replacement**. In the vast majority of patients with advanced arthritis, all three compartments of the knee are affected.

So this has been a basic look at the structures of the knee, but what makes it work? The muscles of the body are the prime movers of the joints. In the case of the knee, your thigh muscles do the bulk of the work. Recall that muscles are connected to bones through tendons (**See Figure 2.6**). In the front of the thigh is a group of four large muscles collectively called the quadriceps muscles (**See Figure 2.7, page 34**). When these muscles contract they cause your knee to straighten. Here's how it works: First, the quadriceps muscles exert a force on the quadriceps tendon. This, in turn, will pull on the top of the patella. The patella then transfers that tension force to the patellar ligament. The patellar ligament then pulls the tibia up to a straight position. This series of connections and muscle contractions make up the extensor mechanism of the knee (**See Figure 2.6**). During this action, the patella acts like the fulcrum of a lever and magnifies the force exerted by the quadriceps muscles giving you more power in knee extension.

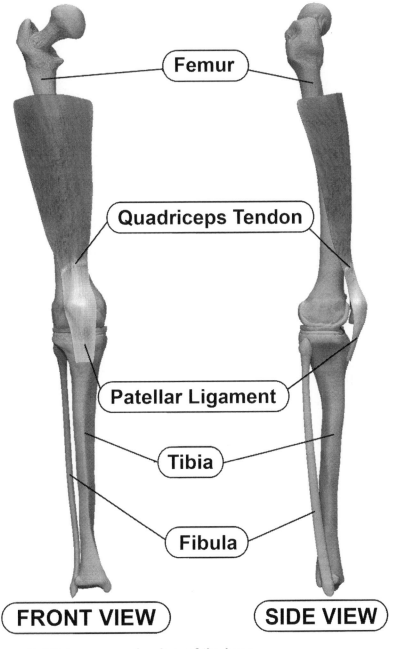

Figure 2.6 Extensor mechanism of the knee

To flex the knee, the muscles behind the thigh are used. A group of three large muscles collectively called the *hamstrings* connect to the back and side of the tibia in numerous locations (**See Figure 2.7**). The net effect is that when the hamstrings contract they bend (flex) the knee by pulling on the back of the tibia. Because the hamstrings and quadriceps have opposite actions on the knee they are referred to as *antagonists*, meaning that when one tightens, the one on the other side of the bone loosens and vice versa.

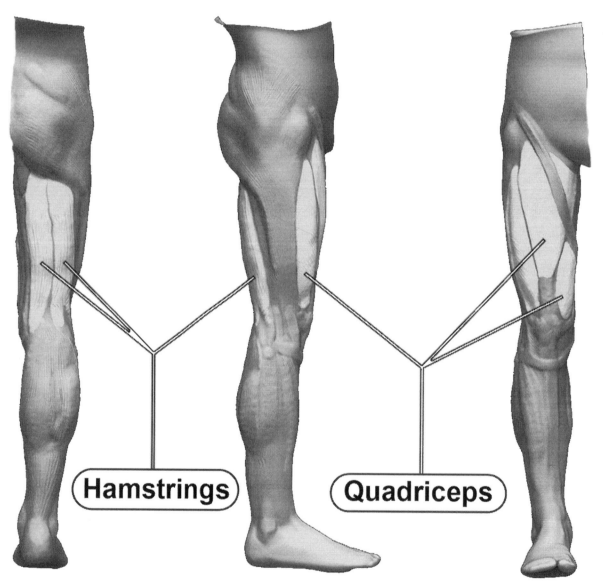

Figure 2.7 Major muscle groups of the thigh

Hip Joint Anatomy

Ok, now let's talk about hip anatomy. Because of the shape of the hip joint, hip anatomy is simpler than that of the knee. The hip, like the knee, is also a highly mobile synovial joint. Recall that synovial joints have cartilage on the ends of the bones and lubricating fluid within the joint which is held in place by a thick capsule. That's about where the similarities end, though. While the knee is often described as a hinge-like joint, the hip is more adequately described as a ball-and-socket joint (**See Figures 2.9 and 2.11, pages 36 and 37**).

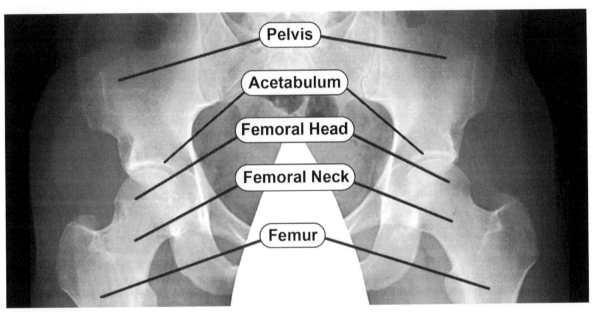

Figure 2.8 X-ray of pelvic anatomy

The "ball" at the top of the femur is called the *femoral head* (**See Figures 2.8 and 2.9**). Under normal circumstances, it is nearly perfectly spherical. The surface of the femoral head is covered with smooth articular cartilage. There is a large ligament within the hip joint that connects the femoral head to the socket. This ligament is called the *ligamentum teres*. Although it does act to help stabilize the hip (keep it from popping out of joint), its main function was as a source of blood supply (during the early years of hip development) as a child. The femoral head is attached to the rest of the femur through a segment of bone called the *femoral neck*.

The capsule of the hip joint attaches to the base of the femoral neck. The femoral neck sees more stress on a daily basis than almost any other bone in the body (**See Figure 2.9**), which is why broken hips are so common. All of the weight of the body is passed through the pelvis into the hip joints and through the femoral necks. At the base of the femoral neck are two protrusions on the femur, one large and one small. These are called the *greater and lesser trochanters* (**See Figure 2.11**), and they serve as attachment points for major tendons. These attachment points, and the muscles that attach to them, are important for hip strength and function.

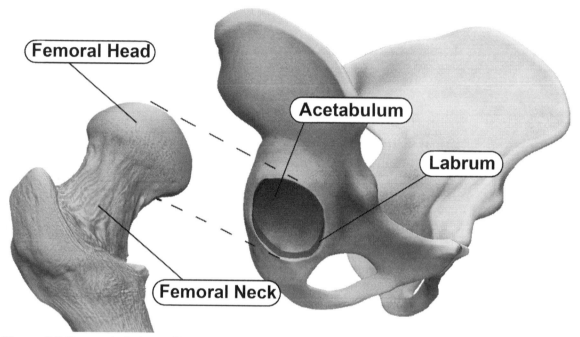

Figure 2.9 Separated view of hip anatomy

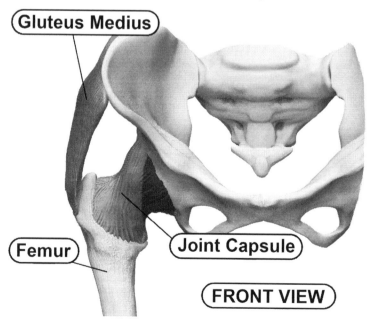

Figure 2.10 Pelvis, gluteus medius and joint capsule

The socket portion of the hip joint is called the *acetabulum* (**See Figure 2.9**). This translates to "vinegar cup" in Latin. The acetabulum is almost perfectly spherical in shape and normally is an exact complement to the femoral head. Along with the articular cartilage over the surface of the bone, there is also a circular cartilage at the edge of the acetabulum called the *labrum*, which helps to form the seal between the femoral head and the acetabulum.

The hip joint is considered an "intrinsically stable" joint, meaning that the bone's shape is the main factor keeping it from dislocating. This is in contrast to the knee joint which relies on numerous ligaments and tendons to keep it from dislocating. Although there is a strong capsule surrounding the hip joint (**See Figure 2.11**), and there is some ligamentous support for the hip as well, most of its stability is due to the shape of the ball-and-socket itself.

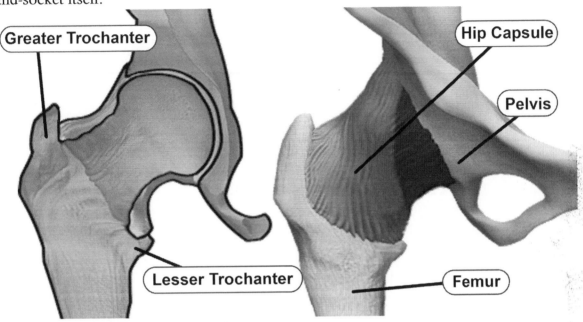

Figure 2.11 Cutaway view of hip anatomy

There are numerous muscles that attach around the hip joint. The most important in terms of strength and gait is the gluteus medius muscle (**See Figure 2.10**) that attaches to the greater trochanter of the femur (**See Figure 2.11**). This muscle is also referred to as the *main abductor* of the hip because of the action it imparts on the hip. Abduction is the act of moving your leg and thigh directly out to the side. If the gluteus medius is weak or damaged, the result is usually a characteristic limp after surgery. For that reason, most of the surgical approaches for hip replacement surgery avoid injury to the gluteus medius muscle and its attachment. This is also the muscle that is mainly targeted for strengthening during rehabilitation after hip replacement surgery.

Lastly, there are conditions that will cause the hip to become less stable. A common cause of instability and arthritis is *hip dysplasia*. This is a condition in which the cup (**See Figures 2.9 and 2.11**) is not formed completely during development in the womb. As a result, the ball does not have a deep enough socket to sit in, and therefore falls out of the socket—or shifts within the socket—very easily. Another common cause for hip dislocation is trauma. In a severe fall or motor vehicle accident, the socket can be broken and/or the ball can be forced out of the joint.

Arthritis

So what goes wrong when you have osteoarthritis? A few things can happen that cause pain in joints. The bottom line is that the hip and knee joints are like well-oiled machines, but because they are so precise, they are also susceptible to problems if there are small changes (or even moderate deterioration). A fine Swiss watch would not tolerate a speck of loose dirt or a slightly bent gear and neither will your joints in the long term. For example, a *fracture* (broken bone) that involves the joint can damage the articular cartilage and create arthritis because the joint surfaces will no longer align perfectly.

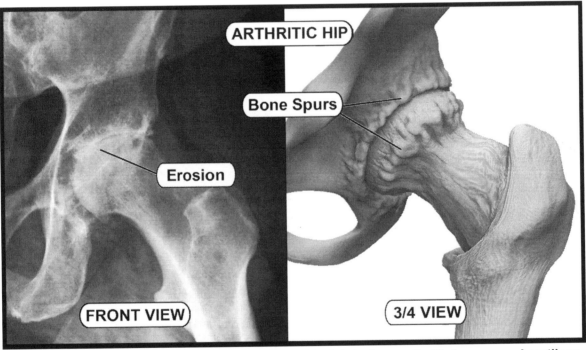

Figure 2.12 X-ray and illustration of degenerated hip joint where arthritis has caused cartilage erosion, shape distortion, and bone spurs

You can certainly damage the cartilage of the joint without breaking the bone as well. If there is damage to a ligament whose job is important to stabilizing the joint, or if you dislocate a joint in an accident, it can become loose and this will cause arthritis because the bones will shift excessively and create wear and/or shearing of the cartilage. Also, the effects of age, genetics, weight, and lifestyle can simply wear the cartilage to the point that it's no longer effective (**See Figures 2.12 and 2.13**). As we discussed above, hip joints can sometimes be misshapen from birth in such a way that the cartilage wears more quickly over the average lifespan as well.

Worn cartilage gets thinner, frays, and swells with water to the point that it is no longer an effective cushion. When this occurs tissues in and around the joint become irritated and painful. In addition, the joint's fluid can also lose its viscosity (becoming more watery) and therefore doesn't lubricate the moving parts as well as it should.

You may also get small pieces of cartilage or bone that break off inside the joint, causing locking or catching of the joint—this is an indicator of joint degeneration. Moreover, even if the joint doesn't catch or lock, these unwanted events obviously distort the normal shape of the joint in it's various anatomical components. Osteoarthritis can also cause bone spurs to form (**See Figures 2.12 and 2.13**), which can limit range of motion when the spurs pinch and grind on the ligaments, tendons, and/or bones of the joint.

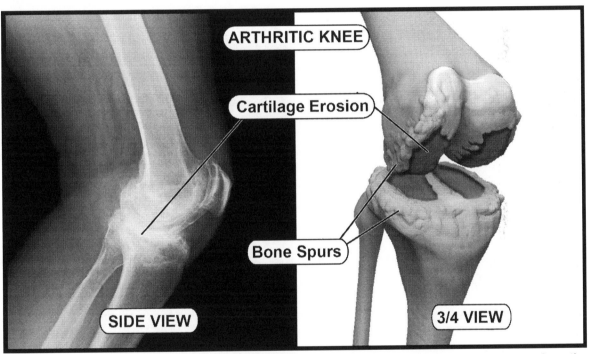

Figure 2.13 X-ray and illustration of degenerated knee joint where arthritis has caused carti-lage erosion, shape distortion, and bone spurs

You can also develop a deformity—especially of the knee—in severe cases of arthritis. For example, if the cartilage on the inner aspect of the knee wears out faster than that on the outer aspect, you will develop a bowed knee. This is the most common deformity seen in osteoarthritis of the knee. When this happens it accelerates the arthritis because the bowing deformity interferes with uniform weight distribution across the knee's surfaces.

Why does arthritis hurt so much? Our bones are not static chunks of calcium, but are living, dynamic structures within each of us which support us and give us our ability to move, run, jump, and play. They have a vast and rich network of blood vessels going in and through them and even have special marrow inside which creates our blood cells. Our joints have nerves around them, which register pain. When the knee or hip joint is deteriorating from osteoarthritis, or injured in some way, the nerves around that joint do their duty to let you know about the problem. Pain is the body's natural reaction to injury and nature's way of telling us that something is wrong.

This was a very brief and simplified description of some very complex structures and mechanisms. We have touched on the major relevant anatomy and physiology of the hip and knee joints and what happens in arthritis. Use this information as a starting point when you discuss things with your surgeon. If you know what I have described above, you'll be far ahead of your peers in your ability to talk with your surgeon and understand her language.

Ask to see your X-rays and have the surgeon describe what her findings are. Often it is apparent, even to laypeople, when they see their X-rays that something is amiss. If your surgeon has a model of the hip or knee joint (and most do), then ask her to show you the model and specifically what areas of your joint are affected. I find that showing my patients their X-rays and going over their condition with the models in my office are valuable aids to their understanding.

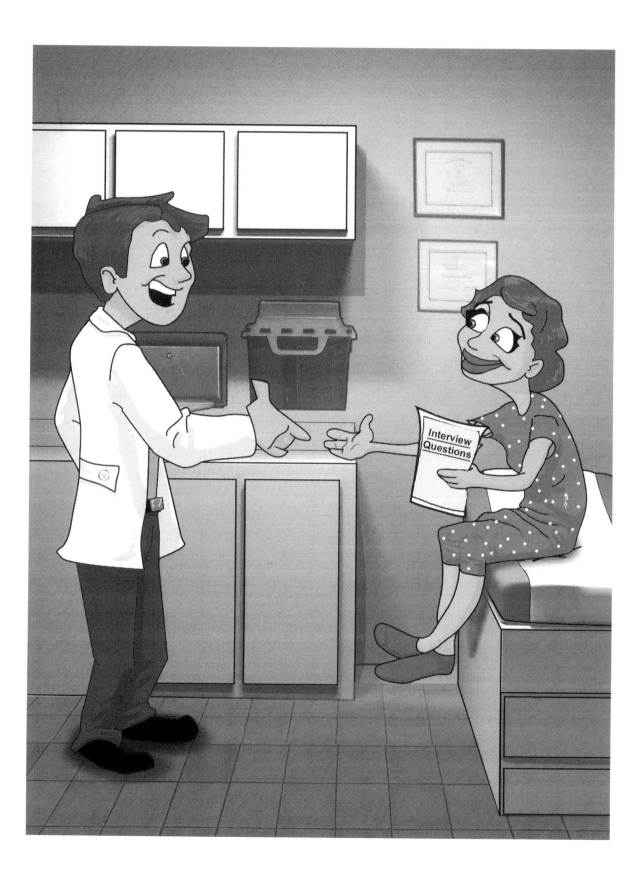

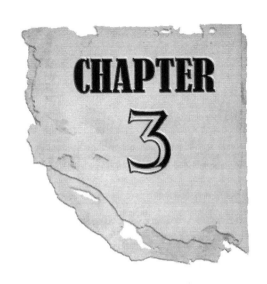

How to go About Selecting a Surgeon: Do's and Don'ts

CHAPTER 3

by Dr. Hugate

One of the many great things about living in this day and age is that we have an abundance of qualified medical specialists in every field of medicine and surgery—and they're very good at what they do! Citizens all over the world now have access to advanced treatment options administered by well-trained, compassionate, and competent providers. This is especially true in the field of orthopedic surgery. I have friends and colleagues from all over the world who are wonderful surgeons, do outstanding work, and stay at the forefront of their respective fields.

I introduce this chapter by saying this because I want you to realize that you have *choices* when deciding who your surgeon should be. Orthopedic surgeons are not in short supply in most parts of the developed world. Here we will briefly discuss how to make the choice of surgeon that best fits you and your family. Don't take this decision lightly. Even if your joint replacement goes perfectly well you may be seeing this surgeon for routine follow-ups for the rest of your life. Consequently, it's very important to choose wisely. Here are a few helpful tips from my perspective as a board certified Orthopedic Surgeon. Because I live and work in the USA, some of this information will be United States specific, but much of it will be universally applicable.

Seek Referrals

Most often the first surgeon you see is introduced to you through your Primary Care Provider (PCP). Once your PCP has deemed that you may be a candidate for hip or knee replacement surgery, he typically has one or two orthopedic surgeons to whom he sends his patients for initial evaluation. This referral pattern can be due to a number of factors. The PCPs typically have a good "pulse" on the local medical community and have a good sense of which orthopedic surgeons do good work and have happy patients. Referrals can also be made from a PCP to an orthopedic surgeon who may be in his insurance "network." By this I mean a network of acceptable physicians for referral as preferred providers for your insurance company. Don't be afraid to ask your PCP why he is referring you to this particular doctor and don't be afraid to ask for more than one recommendation. Your PCP is your best advocate and will point you in the right direction. But consider this referral a starting point rather than a definitive, ending point in your search for the right surgeon.

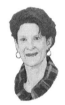

Campone's Comment: I want to echo Dr. Hugate's recommendation. Surgery is serious and significant, and the ability to trust your new surgeon is a critical factor in establishing an expectation of a positive outcome. Because I had a long-time, trusting relationship with my family physician, I was able to transfer that trust to the surgeon he recommended. That did not stop me from drawing my own conclusions after meeting the recommended doctor and listening to my gut instincts as well as his responses to my questions. I also had my "scientist husband" come to the initial meeting with the surgeon and (later on) offer me a "second opinion" of my initial assessment of the doctor I chose. I did ask many of the questions that Dr. Hugate notes in the chapter below. I also looked closely at the overall operation of the doctor's office. Was the reception area welcoming and comfortable? Did staff greet us respectfully and warmly? Were appointments kept on time or was the doctor always running late? How was communication managed? Overall, is there a tone of a well-run team operating in alignment to support the patient's well-being? ~*~

You should also talk to your friends. Many people considering joint replacement surgery are in social circles with others who have undergone this kind of surgery themselves. What better way to get feedback on which surgeons to see and which to avoid? In fact, most of my referrals come through word-of-mouth from prior patients. Take your friends who have had joint replacement surgery out to lunch and spend some time with them. This will give you quality time to catch up, and you can inquire about their experience and ask for wisdom and advice.

Ask them how they felt about their surgeon and their surgery.

- ❏ How did they feel about the hospital?
- ❏ Do they get enough "face time" with their surgeon?
- ❏ How does their hip or knee feel now?
- ❏ Would they do it all over again?
- ❏ And if they wouldn't, what would they change?
- ❏ Do they feel that their surgeon cares about them, or does the surgeon simply act like a skilled technician?
- ❏ What are their surgeon's best and worst attributes?
- ❏ What would your friends change (if they could) about their experience?

This is all valuable feedback from people who have been through it. If you're able to get recommendations by word of mouth, put those surgeons on your list of potentials.

Do Your Own Research

There is also an ever-expanding group of local blogs and support groups available on the World Wide Web for people who have gone through hip or knee replacement surgery. Here you will see the good, the bad, and the ugly. If you see a pattern of praise and affection for a surgeon, consider adding him or her to your list of potential surgeons and then follow up. You have nothing to lose aside from the monetary cost of a few co-pays to visit that surgeon. This is money and time well spent. There are a number of commercial sites on the World Wide Web which allow former and current patients to "rank their doctors." These are another source of information, but be cautious about how you interpret them. Overwhelmingly, people who choose to rate their doctor do so because they've had a bad experience and wish to *punish* the surgeon's reputation. The general rule-of-thumb is that while a happy patient may tell two or three friends about their good experiences, an unhappy patient will tell at least *ten* friends (or anybody who will listen) about a bad experience. This bias is often reflected in the so-called doctor ranking websites.

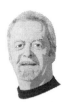

Holland's Comment: As to blogs and such on the World Wide Web: there is an inherent problem with almost everything you see posted—namely, there is little or no accountability. A blogger can canonize (that is, hand out blessings) or demonize a physician (that is, roast her on a spit) depending on his mood at the time, and nobody else can call him on it except to post more ratings to that same blog. Eventually the truth gets buried in the avalanche of muckraking. Think of all this as "online gossip" and you'll see it for what it is. Granted, physicians have their difficult moments like all of us, and no physician is a saint. However, you can rest assured that eventually, those physicians who are closer to the other end of the spectrum will be institutionally weeded out. Unfortunately, you'll seldom hear from the great bulk of us out here in the world who have had 100 percent positive outcomes. Most busy people are quite happy to simply move on with their lives and therefore do not contribute their experiences to online web blogs or handbooks like this. ~*~

I would strongly caution against using an orthopedic implant manufacturer's websites to choose your surgeon. These sites can be less than objective and here's why: the manufacturers who produce hip and knee implants are part of an enormous industry, and this is very big business. So the implant companies employ a number of marketing strategies to improve sales. As an example, let's consider a fictional implant company called **"Implants For You and Me"** (aka IFYM). If Dr. X tends to use the IFYM knee replacement system, then the IFYM website will tout Dr. X as the best surgeon since sliced bread. Is it because Dr. X is a really good knee replacement surgeon? Perhaps, but more likely it's because IFYM knows that every knee replacement candidate who sees Dr. X is another potential sale for them. This is not to say that Dr. X isn't a great surgeon, but simply being mentioned on the IFYM website should be taken in the proper context.

The same may be true for the advertisement of so-called "cutting-edge" techniques. Still using our hypothetical company (IFYM), let's say that they develop a new "minimally invasive" technique to reduce the size of a hip replacement incision and this new technique requires the use of tools, instruments, retractors, and aiming devices only available through IFYM. Again, on the IFYM website you'll find that Dr. X is one of only a handful of surgeons in the world who is trained in this cutting-edge technique. The implication is that you'd be a fool not to have your joint replacement done by Dr. X using IFYM equipment, implants, and procedures. Right? Not necessarily! The answer here is the same as above: IFYM obviously has a vested interest in promoting their techniques and products in whatever way they can, so more information is needed outside of their commercial marketing silo. Take my advice: you're better off doing your *due diligence* as outlined throughout this handbook.

Please understand that I'm telling you this *not to bash the implant manufacturers*, but to educate you as to their potential perspectives and motivations. Let me clearly state that the major implant companies are superb and without their tireless efforts at design, development of materials, innovation, and exhaustive testing of their implants we would not have the great outcomes that we do. They are an extremely important part of the medical team and the success of joint replacements is based on the successful design and manufacture of their implants. Without good quality implants, it wouldn't matter how good your medical team—you would do poorly. They just do what any good company does: promote the use of their products. We cannot fault them for that, but neither should we base major decisions about our own health care on their promotional strategies.

Examine Credentials

Once you have a list of potential surgeons for your surgery, the first basic issue to consider is that of qualifications. Is this surgeon qualified to perform your joint replacement surgery? This is typically not an issue in the developed world, but you should still do your due diligence. Fortunately, most countries have a demanding process to earn the credentials to perform surgery. In the United States, the **American Board of Orthopedic Surgery** (ABOS, https://www.abos.org/) oversees a rigorous board certification process in which prospective surgeons must go through a number of academic and performance hoops to earn the title of "Board Certified Orthopedic Surgeon."

In order to be certified by the ABOS, an individual must have completed college (4+ years), medical school (4+ years), a surgical internship (1 year), an orthopedic surgical residency (4 years), and completed 2 years of satisfactory clinical practice. In addition they must pass a two-part examination process that culminates in a face-to-face defense and academic discussion with world experts (on various fields in orthopedic surgery) about how they treat their patients. Some surgeons even go on to do "fellowships." Fellowships are additional years of training at a more advanced level in a certain subspecialty within orthopedics. All of this is a long-winded way to say that your best bet toward ensuring that an orthopedic surgeon has *basic* qualifications in the USA is to ensure that they're ABOS certified.

The state licensing board is generally a good source of information on whether a surgeon is ABOS certified. This can be discovered through direct contact with the ABOS as well.

However, ABOS certification is not *all* you should look at. This certifies that the doctor is competent in *orthopedic surgery* but not necessarily in *joint replacement surgery*. You see, there are some orthopedic surgeons who don't perform (or perform very few) joint replacements. You will want a surgeon who regularly performs joint replacements. Joint replacement surgery is also referred to as "adult reconstruction," so you may see this wording, but the terms are synonymous. Most orthopedic surgeons advertise their specialties, but if it's not clear to you what the surgeon specializes in, simply call her office and ask how many hip or knee replacements does Dr. X perform annually? Research has shown the obvious: the more of any procedure that a doctor performs, the better she gets. If an orthopedic surgeon performs less than ten hip or knee replacements per year, she is likely to be less adept at performing these procedures than one who performs 100+ joint replacements per year.

Next, take a look at the surgeon's practice history and background. In the age of the World Wide Web, it's fast, easy, and cheap to do your own "background check" on any prospective surgeon. There are a number of commercial and government on-line resources that will allow you to search the background of the doctors you're considering. Information that can be found on-line includes board certification status, state licensing, licensing board reprimands or punishments, criminal background, malpractice lawsuits, or any behavioral or substance abuse issues. Many surgeons also post their Curriculum Vitae (essentially the surgeon's resume) online as well, which will give you insight as to their training, research activities, publications, leadership roles, and so on. Remember that CVs emphasize the positive, so simply reading a prospective surgeon's CV will (potentially) tell only half of the story. Also be aware that if you discover a surgeon has been sued, that doesn't mean he's a bad doctor. Unfortunately, America is a litigious society, and therefore lawsuits are all too common. So don't be surprised if every doctor you look up has had lawsuits filed against him at some time. The key is how many of those suits were thrown out versus successfully litigated against the doctor. Remember, surgeons are humans—just like you. So don't be surprised if you find some less-than-flattering facts about any surgeon during your research. Try to be fair in your assessment and look for patterns of struggles rather than isolated instances.

Once you've done your homework, narrow your list of potential surgeons to two or three. If your research is good, that should be enough to get you to the right doctor without breaking the bank. The next step is obvious: make some appointments! As you do, make note of how friendly the staff is and how helpful they are. They should take steps and possibly do additional checks to ensure that the physician is a *preferred provider* with your insurance carrier. Otherwise, you may get stuck with the entire bill for the visit. Make note of how long a wait there is to see the doctor, as this will give you some indication as to her accessibility. Ask specifically whether you'll see the doctor or her assistant. Some surgeons have their assistants do most of the office work and actually visit their patients in the office on the rare occasion. This is not to say they are bad doctors, but if your goal is to have more face time with the surgeon, you may be disappointed in this model of practice. If the doctor's office is in a less convenient location, *make the trip anyway*! You do *not* want to make a decision about which doctor performs your surgery based on the surgeon who has offices closest to your home. If you find the right surgeon, it will be well worth the time invested in driving.

At the Doctor's Office

Now, for the actual visit, consider it an interview and you're the boss. I don't mean that you should be cocky or overly demanding, but use this time to size up the surgeon and determine whether your interpersonal relations are a good fit, and whether *this* is the doctor who gets to be your surgeon.

Consider the following questions:

- ❏ Did the surgeon take the time to explain your condition?
- ❏ Did she go over all potential options?
- ❏ Did she discuss the potential risks of the recommended treatment?
- ❏ Did you feel that the doctor cared about you?
- ❏ Ask to look at your X-rays and ask if there are any models of the joint you're speaking about. Many offices have plastic demonstration models of various joints to help point out issues and to help show you what the issues are.
- ❏ Where can the doctor perform the operation (that is, at what hospitals or surgical centers)?
- ❏ How many hip or knee replacements do they perform in an average year?
- ❏ Who is the *second* best joint replacement surgeon in town?

This last question from the checklist above (about who is second best) is somewhat loaded because all surgeons feel as if they are the best in town. You therefore might get a chuckle from your doctor out of this one. What this question will do, though, is give you another name for a potential second or third opinion. These are all great questions to ask the doctor.

I wouldn't recommend asking the surgeon what her complication rate is. Chances are you won't get an accurate response. That's like asking a father who his least favorite child is. We surgeons tend to be biased in favor of ourselves. Make no mistake, you can't be a surgeon and jump through all those hoops and endure all those years of training without emerging with an ego. True, some egos are bigger than others, but any surgeon who denies that he has an ego is lying, and you should turn around and run away as fast as your bad joints will take you! It's a fact of life. Complication rates are better determined through the other means we've discussed above. If you want to ask the question just to see what reaction you get, OK—just remember there's inherent (unconscious) bias in the answer.

I would also recommend that you avoid getting into complex discussions with your doctor regarding the brand of implant to be used for your hip or knee replacement. We surgeons realize that the general public is peppered with biased information from various sources and we're getting more requests for a specific brand of hip or knee replacement implant than ever before. I think if you're a younger, more active patient, it's reasonable to ask the surgeon if she uses a *different* implant for that population of patients (and why?), but brand name discussions are generally not fruitful. The bottom line is that your surgeon uses the same group of implants on a daily basis because, in her hands, her patients have done well. She's familiar with that brand's sizing and surgical instrumentation. This familiarity makes for a smoother and more successful surgery. If your surgeon changed the brand of implant at every request it would force her into using systems she's not familiar with and it could potentially end up with less-than-desirable results. Inquiring in general terms is OK, but don't try to force your surgeon out of her comfort zone by demanding that a certain brand be used for your joint replacement.

Now, repeat that process for the other one or two candidate surgeons on your list unless you're completely satisfied with the first one. You should also mention to the doctors you consult that you're considering obtaining a second opinion. This is a litmus test of sorts. If the surgeon is offended or takes exception to a second opinion, consider that a red flag. In my opinion, no confident, competent surgeon should be offended or feel threatened by a second opinion.

I don't recommend that you make the decision to have hip or knee replacement while you're in the doctor's office. Take some time to think about it—mull it over. If you feel pressure from the surgeon or their staff to schedule the surgery right then and there, then consider that a red flag too! Remember this is an elective surgery and there is no urgency. Many people won't purchase a car or house until they've "slept on it," so why make a hasty decision regarding choice of surgery or a surgeon? Take as much time as you need to feel that you've made the right choice.

I hope this plan as I've laid it out helps. If I were in need of a joint replacement, this is exactly what I would do. If you follow this advice, you'll most likely end up in the right hands—literally!

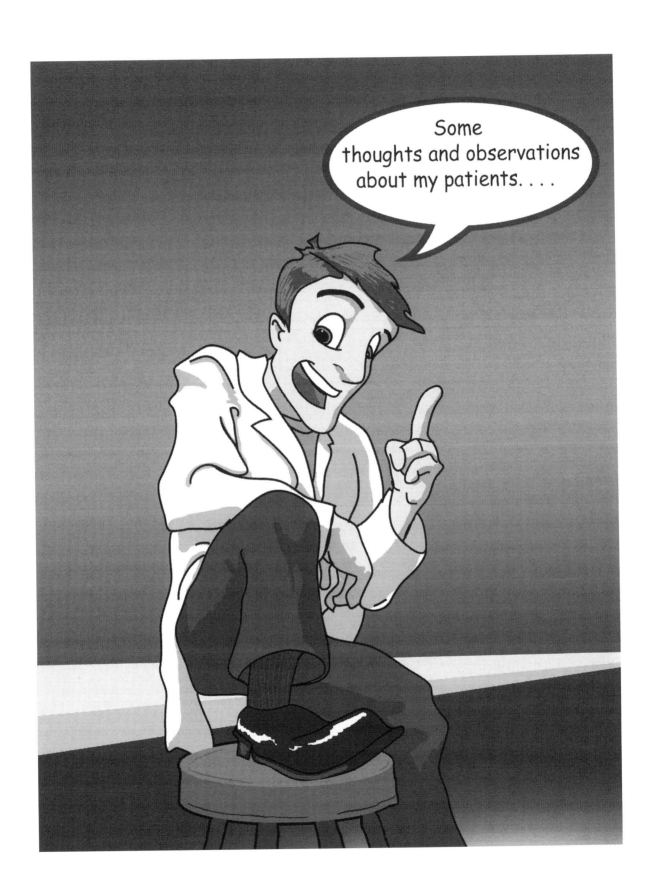

Thoughts and Observations about Patients

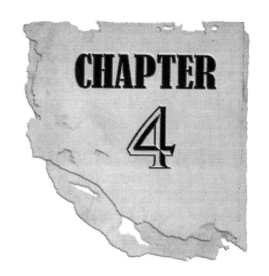

CHAPTER 4

by Dr. Hugate

Patients, like doctors, come in all shapes and sizes with an endless number of inter-esting personalities and medical complexities. No two patients are the same and this what makes my profession interesting and challenging—and why I love what I do. Let's say, for the sake of discussion, that I have two patients who come to see me with painful, arthritic knees. They're roughly the same age and health status overall. Both elect to have their knees replaced and their surgeries go well. They should both do great, right? The real answer is, "Not always." There are a number of moving parts in the process of total joint replacement and one of the most important moving parts is *you*, the patient! While your surgeon bears great responsibility in performing your hip or knee replacement in a technically proficient manner and managing your medical and surgical issues, the vast majority of the work and effort required to make a joint replacement a success falls on the patient's shoulders. I often tell my patients the morning after their surgery, "The easy part is over... now the *real* work begins."

So let's take some time now to go over what I've observed in my years of taking care of patients. During that time I've been privileged to care for thousands of people and learned something from each. What I intend to discuss in this chapter is which "patient specific traits" are associated with successful outcomes and which ones are not.

Health Maintenance

Let's start with your health maintenance. While we can't always pick what health problems we have, most of us can certainly decide to keep up with our health maintenance.

There's no question that the healthier you are when you go into surgery, the healthier you'll be coming out, and the better your chances for success. A doctor's worst nightmare is a patient who never sees his Primary Care Provider (PCP), or doesn't even have one, and has multiple medical problems that have been developing unchecked for years.

Attention to your overall health is very important. It reduces your risk for anesthetic and surgical complications and vastly improves your ability to rehabilitate after surgery. Your PCP is a wizard when it comes to medically managing chronic illnesses and keeping you in the best health possible despite whatever conditions you may have. Heart conditions, diabetes, blood pressure issues, thyroid issues, high cholesterol, and a slew of other chronic medical conditions all need to be well monitored and controlled under your PCP's supervision before you consider having a joint replacement. A weight loss effort or a smoking cessation plan (if necessary) should also be considered well before surgery and your PCP is your best resource in helping come up with a plan for these important issues. The time and money you spend on getting your annual checkups will pay tremendous dividends whether or not you decide to have joint replacement surgery.

Support

The next category of patients who tend to do well are those with support. Family, friends, clergy—you name it—anyone you can trust and confide in and who simply cares about you. There's no question in my mind that patients who have someone accompany them through this journey do better in every way. Moreover, this companion should be included in the journey and decision-making process *prior* to the decision to have surgery. Having a supportive friend or family member there with you when you visit your surgeon gives you another set of ears and eyes to hear, see, and help you *understand* what the surgeon is saying. You can bounce ideas off of him or her, or discuss the advice you received at the surgeon's office prior to committing to any course of treatment.

Invariably, patients with supportive friends or family members at their bedside tend to get better care while in the hospital because they can help bring your issues and needs to the attention of the busy hospital staff. Supportive individuals are invaluable during the postoperative outpatient rehabilitation both in terms of emotional support and practical support—making sure you get to physical therapy and doctor appointments on time, taking your medications, ensuring that you keep up with your home exercise regimen, and so on. There are few things that sadden me like a patient who shows up for his appointments and surgery alone. In some cases, the patients simply may not have enough support, but I would say that in the majority of cases, these patients have supportive family members or friends but *choose* not to include them in their care. Maybe they feel as if they don't want to burden them or they feel capable of handling things on their own. This is a mistake in my opinion. Make an effort to include someone else in your care, and you will not be sorry!

Campone's Comment: Caregiving is an essential element of building and strengthening relationships, whether these are marital relationships or friendships. My husband's role as cheerleader, nurse, and exercise-coach was invaluable in supporting my recovery. It gave him an opportunity to express forms of caring that are not an ordinary part of our day-to-day relationship. Friends who volunteered to take me walking benefitted from the exercise and fresh air as well. Most people have an innate desire to do good; giving them an opportunity to fulfill that desire is a win-win situation. ~*~

Realistic Expectations

In addition, patients with *realistic expectations* tend to do better than those with unrealistic expectations. What do I mean by this? One of my mentors during training used to tell me, "Being a good surgeon is first and foremost about setting realistic expectations." and I believe he was right. Consider two hypothetical patients: Mr. Jones and Mr. Smith. Mr. Jones has had debilitating arthritis for years and simply wants to be able to walk without pain and play with his small grandchildren. Mr. Smith, on the other hand, also has painful arthritis, but his main goal is to get back to championship level racquetball competition. They both get the same operation and have the same outcome (no pain and full range of motion). However, because of the limitations on high-demand activities with joint replacements, Mr. Smith is unable to get back to his aggressive racquetball competitions and is therefore disappointed in his new knee. Mr. Jones, however, can play all day with his three-year-old grandson and is entirely satisfied with his new knee. This is usually due to a failure on the part of the surgeon to communicate well enough prior to surgery what patients should expect and what level of activity they can expect to return to. A joint replacement does a great job of relieving pain and deformity. However, the replaced joint will never be *normal* again, even if the operation is entirely successful.

Holland's Comment: It's been more than two years since Dr. Hugate put the new knee in my right leg. There are still times after a hike when it's a bit uncomfortable, but I rub some analgesic gel on it and it's fine—and while I'm on the hike I don't even think about it. Contrast this with when I used to try to hike just before my knee replacement. I once had knee pain so bad I feared I'd have to have my wife walk out and call in the Alpine Rescue Team! I had walked about three miles in and on the way back out, coming down the trail, the knee began to burn with excruciating pain. Only a half-mile after turning back, I was using my six-foot walking stick as a crutch.

Now I walk like a pro and I hike as far as I want! My limitations are minimal. For example, I have reduced resistance to the winter weather and I tend to avoid kneeling down for reasons we cover later in our handbook. Dr. Hugate told me I had to be sensible: no jumping off the pickup tailgate, no aggressive basketball, no high-impact running. Well, what the heck—it's been years since I did those things anyway. ~*~

There are limitations imparted on a patient once their joint is replaced. We'll go over these limitations in more detail later in the handbook, but impact activities (such as aggressive racquetball) tend to "wear out" the joint replacements much quicker and can loosen the joint replacement parts. For that reason, running (or any high-impact activity) is not recommended after knee or hip replacement. Abrupt twisting, turning, and cutting type activities are generally not handled well by joint replacements either. Had Mr. Smith known and accepted these limitations prior to his surgery, he'd be more likely to perceive his outcome as favorable.

Play an Active Role in Your Care

Patients who take an active role in their care have better outcomes as well. Being a patient in this day and age is *not* a passive experience—nor should it be. It's *not* like taking a clunky old car to the mechanic and dropping it off for repair. No, having total joint replacement surgery is more than this. The fact that you're reading this handbook is a good sign. It means you have engaged yourself in the process, and the knowledge you gain will empower you to make the right decisions and do the right things. That knowledge also changes the dynamic between you and your doctor. In the *old days* of medical practice, patients would come in to see the doctor and the doctor would say, "Here's what you need to have done," and the patient would say, "Ok, doc. Whatever you say." It was all very paternalistic and one-sided. Times are changing, and we doctors expect and encourage patients to question and examine what we're advising them to do. It's rare that I tell a patient that she really *needs* to have something done. More often than not, I give patients the information they need to make the right decision *for themselves*. This helps invest my patients in their own care and everyone is happier—and far healthier—in the end.

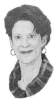 **Campone's Comment:** I second Dr. Hugate's affirmation. My hip surgeon actively encouraged questions and was perfectly willing to spend as much time as I required making sure I understood his answers. As someone who's very curious by nature (and training), I wanted (and needed) to:

- Have X-rays explained,
- Understand the sequence of events in the course of the surgery,
- Explore the various factors that are generally involved in the development of arthritis,
- Understand the role of family genetics,
- Learn about the doctor's experience and results,
- And, clarify the roles (and qualifications) of each of the people on his team.

As noted above, I also looked closely at how he and his team members interacted, which reinforces Dr. Hugate's point about the surgeon's ability to effectively coordinate his time in support of my surgery. Every patient is unique and so every surgery is unique, and it's important that the surgeon and his team are able to be responsive to the individual—not just produce an assembly-line, surgical routine. ~*~

Compliance

Compliant patients likewise have better outcomes. What is a compliant patient? Well, it's one who *listens to the doctor's instructions* before, during, and after surgery and follows them with determination, good judgment, and diligence. Seems like a no-brainer, right? But for a variety of reasons (with both patients and doctors at fault) this doesn't always happen. Maybe instructions weren't given or weren't made clear enough. Sometimes the patient hears the instruction but chooses not to abide for whatever reason. I had a patient once who had his knee replaced, and the surgery went great. He was discharged from the hospital with the usual instructions and prescriptions and, of course, one of those prescriptions was for physical therapy to regain his range of motion. Unfortunately he had a friend who had a TKR and this friend told my patient that physical therapy wasn't very important, and he could easily save him some money by simply showing him what needed to be done at home. Six weeks passed and this patient was unable to fully straighten the knee. I won't go into detail here, but this specific issue (around physical therapy) is critical and creates long-term, debilitating problems. Have you ever tried walking on a knee that won't straighten? It's exhausting and painful.

The bottom line is you're paying your doctor "big bucks" to give you the right advice—so take it. That's not to say that you shouldn't ask questions or engage your surgeon if you don't understand an instruction. If you're not sure about something, call the office and speak to the surgeon or his assistant. Remember, no two surgeries are the same, so simply having had a TKR before doesn't make anybody an expert. Yes, listen to the advice of those who've had prior knee replacements, but if their advice strays from that given by your surgeon, discuss it with your surgeon before you let it affect your postoperative regimen.

So use this compilation of observations to stack the deck in your favor. Commit to following your surgeon's instructions. Have somebody with you to help you though your journey. Take an active part in understanding what your objectives are and how you intend to achieve them, and in finding the knowledge to make this undertaking successful. My patients who exhibit these traits put themselves in a much better position for an overall, successful experience.

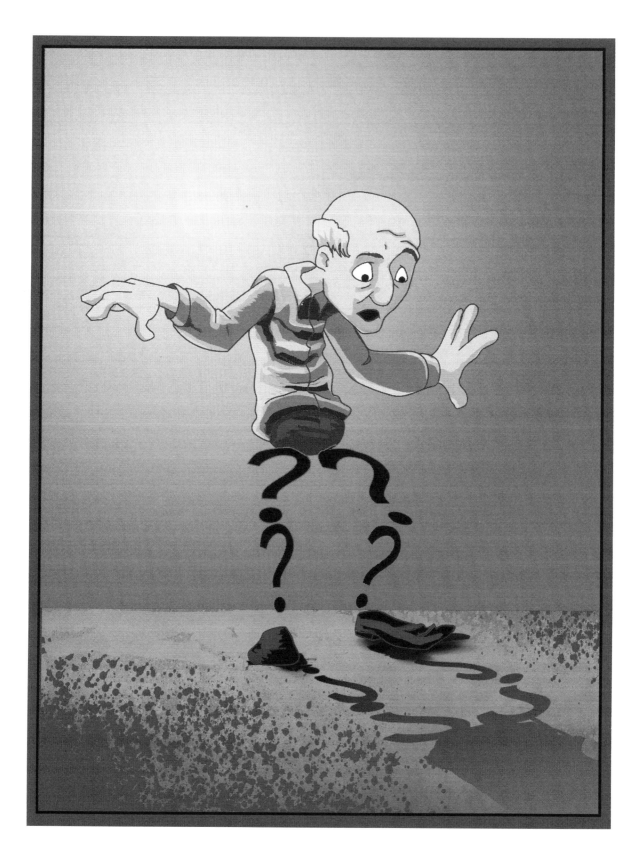

Two Knees or One?

by Dr. Hugate

L et's say you've decided to have knee replacement surgery because your knees are killing you. Nothing works for the pain—not the pills, not the shots, not the weight loss. It's miserable. You can't do the things that make your life worth living. You're relieved that the decision is made and you are ready to move forward with knee replacement. But wait! There's one more question to throw a monkey wrench in the gearbox. Should I have one knee replaced or two? This is a common question I get and I'll outline the reasons why below. As with anything, there are pros and cons to either approach and I'll try to go over the major issues for you to consider here.

Knees are bilaterally symmetric structures on the body (which means you have two of them, and they are mirror images of one another). When you consider the commonly known causes of arthritis, there's no surprise that they can affect both knees. Lifestyle, genetics, weight, and activity are all factors which can work together to wear down *both* knees. For that reason many patients considering knee replacement surgery have arthritis in both knees—hence, the question that titles this chapter. Sure, there is the rare patient who may have injured one knee, or had a severe infection that caused arthritis in only one knee, but many patients with arthritis in one knee will have some degree of arthritis in the other knee as well.

One Knee Replacement versus Two

Let's look at the individual factors and how they stack up when considering having one knee replaced at a time (two operations, separated by at least three months) versus

61

having both knees replaced during the same operation. There are a number of issues to consider when asking the previous question, so let's take look at these and explore who should consider having both knees replaced at once? The first thing I ask my patients is:

Which knee hurts you more?

This question is a great starting point, and it generally elicits one of two responses. The first and most common response is:

While I have pain in both knees, the one knee hurts by far the worst and hurts more often.

These are the vast majority of my patients and are the patients—in my opinion—who should stick with just having one knee replaced. The dynamics are a little tricky here so follow along with me. When a knee is hurting, the natural tendency is to favor the "good knee," shifting most of the work of walking to the knee that hurts the least. This in turn, makes the good knee hurt more. So the pain in the good knee is partly because of some underlying arthritis, but is made *worse* by shifting the weight away from the "bad knee." In these patients, having the bad knee replaced will often improve the symptoms on the good side as well. The reason is that the old pain from the bad knee has been significantly mitigated (possibly even eliminated completely) by the knee replacement, so the good knee is no longer overworked carrying it. Make sense?

If you fall into this category, my advice is to only have the one knee replaced and see how you do. You don't burn any bridges with this approach and you can always decide later to have the other knee replaced if the pain doesn't improve. If this is your situation you need not read further in this chapter.

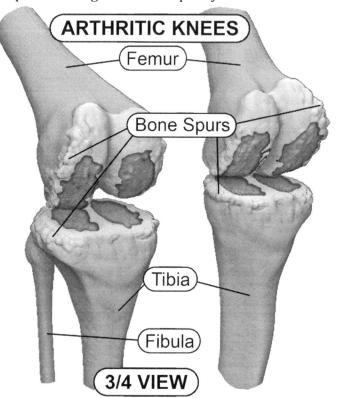

Figure 5.1 Bilateral knees with arthritis

When Both Knees Hurt Equally Bad

The other response that I get much *less* commonly is some version of the following:

Both of my knees hurt equally badly. They tend to take turns flaring up with pain, but both knees flare up an equal amount.

In my opinion, this is the group of patients who meet the *basic* criteria for having both knees replaced. In this group, even if you take the pain out of one knee, the remaining knee's arthritis is so far advanced that it will undoubtedly continue to be a serious problem. Eventually, this knee will likely need to be replaced anyway (**See Figure 5.1**). For these people, we at least explore the option.

There are a number of other issues to consider, of course, and each patient makes his or her own decisions. The real question becomes then:

Should both of the knees be replaced during the same surgery, or should they be replaced during two separate surgeries?

Point-by-point Comparison

Both Knees Replaced at Once versus One at a Time

Anesthetic Considerations

First, let's consider the surgery time in terms of anesthesia risk. A single knee replacement takes the average surgeon about one hour to perform. As you might expect, a bilateral total knee replacement (BTKR) takes about twice that time because you are replacing two knees.

When I do a bilateral knee replacement surgery, I usually start surgery on the knee that is the currently most painful side and complete that side before moving ahead in the operation to the other side. Of course, if the patient is not doing well with the surgery at the end of the first knee replacement, we stop the operation, but usually the patient is doing fine and I continue on to the other knee. So, barring any reason to abort midway through, doing both knees means added operating room (OR) time, which would seem to put you at greater risk, right? Well, not if you consider the fact that if both knees are horribly arthritic, you'll *eventually* need to go on and have the other knee joint replaced in a completely separate operation. So the overall total OR time is not much different when having bilateral knee replacements at one time versus having one knee replaced at a time during separate operations.

What *is* different is this: if you have both knees replaced during one operation, you only go through anesthesia once versus going through anesthesia twice with two separate operations. This is important because undergoing anesthesia is somewhat like taking a plane flight: the most hazardous times are during takeoff (analogous to initiating anesthesia) and landing (analogous to coming out of anesthesia). So theoretically, a single, two-hour flight is safer than two separate one-hour flights. That is, during the two flights you undergo two takeoffs and two landings versus only one of each with a single flight. In that way, with regard to overall OR time and anesthetic risk, the advantage goes to having both knees replaced at the same operation.

Blood Loss

Next let's look at blood loss and the need for transfusion. The risk for needing a blood transfusion is higher in those patients who get both knees replaced at the same time versus those who have one knee replaced at a time in two separate operations. Why? When you undergo bilateral TKR you lose twice the amount of blood than you would during a unilateral TKR. That blood loss can take your blood count down to potentially low levels and therefore require transfusion. On the other hand, if you have both knees replaced at separate times (at least three months apart) you lose half as much blood during the first operation and your body has a chance to build up its blood supply before the next operation. Assuming your blood count is normal by the time you get to your second operation, you very well may never need a transfusion with either surgery. So the advantage here goes to having one knee replaced at a time.

Time Away from Home

How about the hospital stay? The average hospital stay after a single knee replacement is about three days. If you have bilateral knee replacement, you will likely be in the hospital four to five days. But again, you have to consider that the patient undergoing one knee replacement at a time will have two hospital stays, so his or her total hospital stay will be six to seven days, though not all at once. The advantage in hospital days goes to bilateral TKR.

There's another issue to consider, though, and that's the possibility of needing to go to a rehabilitation (rehab) facility versus going home after your single TKR. Think of rehab facilities like inpatient physical therapy. Rehab facilities are NOT nursing homes, because the patients at rehab facilities must be able to participate two to three times per day in rigorous physical therapy. I mention this because if you undergo bilateral TKR, there's a greater possibility that you may need to go to a rehab facility, rather than directly home after your hospital stay. So it's difficult to say which approach will land you more days away from home. Certainly if you look at hospital time alone, the advantage goes to bilateral TKR. But if you consider the possible increased need for rehabilitation after bilateral TKR, you may spend more overall time away from home with the bilateral TKR approach. Lastly on this topic, it's possible you may get to go home after bilateral TKR, but will have extended in-home care from a physical therapist—this will depend on a number of factors, not the least of which is your insurance coverage or financial resources.

Total Rehabilitation Time

What about overall rehabilitation time? This round easily goes to bilateral TKR. Let's go over a hypothetical scenario to illustrate the point. Mr. Green and Mr. White both have knee replacement surgery on January 1st. Mr. Green has one knee replaced and Mr. White has both knees replaced. Both have the usual stay in the hospital after surgery and both go home after the hospital stay. In general, it takes about two months to completely recover from unilateral TKR and about three months to recover from bilateral TKR. Bilateral TKRs take longer to recover from because you literally have no good leg to stand on for the first few weeks. With this being the case, Mr. Green has rehabilitated his knee by the end of February. Meanwhile, Mr. White, having undergone bilateral knee replacements, is not fully rehabilitated until the end of March. The difference here is that Mr. White is done! Both knees are replaced and he can now go about living his life. Mr. Green, on the other hand now has to go back for surgery in mid-March to have his other knee replaced and go through the whole thing again. In this scenario, with both gentlemen having started their operations at the same time, Mr. White will be fully rehabilitated in late March of that year while Mr. White will not be fully rehabilitated until June. There is a clear advantage to bilateral TKR here.

Financial Considerations

Let's look at the financial side of things also. It's important not to ignore this issue. Of course, the particulars of this subject are based on your individual insurance plan, but again, the overall advantage is to BTKR. Why? Consider the fact that if you decide to have two separate TKRs you will have two separate hospital stays and two separate trips to the operating room (OR), and two separate anesthetics as well. You will also likely spend more actual overall time in the hospital if you have the knees done separately. Being an inpatient at the hospital and going to the OR is expensive! When you get that huge bill after your surgery is done remember that the vast majority of that bill is hospital and OR charges—that's where the costs rack up. So if you're able to have both procedures done safely under one hospital stay and during one trip to the OR, you'll reduce your financial burden and that of your insurance company overall. Bilateral TKR wins this round.

Need for Support

Now let's talk about the need for support. While the need for having emotional and practical support from friends and family members is important in both scenarios, those who have both knees replaced at the same time will need a special and more intense level of support. Remember you will have no "good leg" to stand on for at least a few weeks. That means probably needing a wheel chair and certainly needing help with activities of daily living (ADLs) such as shower, meals, toileting, and preparing food. Having a knee replacement is a big operation, but having both knees replaced at the same time is a BIG operation! Make no mistake, you will need someone dedicated to your needs for a few weeks after surgery. The alternative to this is to have a rehab stay (described above) or some sort of at-home, extended caregiver, and at-home physical therapy for three to four weeks after surgery. These home services can help take some burden off of you supporter, but not all.

Holland's Comment: There are more considerations than the purely medical ones. You must consider the practical elements of rehabilitation and recovery and there are other very important stakeholders to keep in mind as well. One of the most important stakeholders in the BTKR journey is your spouse (significant other, or at-home caregiver). As the youngest child, I was the last kid left in town. For the last thirty years of her life I was my mother's primary caregiver when she was sick, in the hospital, or at an extended care facility, and this made me a stakeholder. If she was home, but unable to perform ADLs for any period of time, this impacted both my wife and I and both of our work schedules. With this experience, I can tell you that under no circumstances should you expect your at-home caregiver (whoever that might be) to try and lift you about and support your weight in moving around the house, taking showers, and/or getting in and out of a car. This is a recipe for disaster. ~*~

Risk of Medical Complications

What about potential for medical complications? There is no doubt that having bilateral knee replacements can lead to increased complications. Because of the magnitude of the surgery, it's simply harder on your heart, lungs, and other body systems. It has been shown to be especially dangerous to undergo bilateral TKR for those who are over seventy years old and/or those who have heart or lung issues. Conditions that are seen more commonly in those who undergo bilateral knee replacements are pulmonary embolism (PE, aka blood clot in the lungs), and deep venous thrombosis (DVT, aka blood clot in the legs). Another less common condition known as fatty (or bone-marrow) embolization is increased in those having bilateral knee replacements as well. This is a condition in which fat from the bone marrow gets into the blood stream and deposits in the lungs. If you are at an elevated risk for any of these conditions, avoiding bilateral surgery may seem the best option. On the other hand, you only have to undergo these risks *once* if you have both knees replaced at the same time, whereas having both knees replaced at separate times means you must endure their (lower) surgical risks *twice*.

Summary of Recommendations

So there you have it. Clear as mud, right? There are arguments supporting either approach. Let me summarize with my recommendations based on what I know. If you are a patient who has two painful arthritic knees that are unresponsive to nonsurgical management, and you have knee X-rays consistent with severe arthritis in both knees—*and* if both knees are more or less equally painful—then you are, at a minimum, in the category of patients who could consider having both knees replaced at once (bilateral TKR). Furthermore, I would only consider bilateral TKRs if you are less than seventy years of age and have no significant heart or lung problems. In addition, I offer bilateral TKRs only to well-motivated patients with an excellent support system in place. I would *not* perform bilateral TKRs on anyone who would refuse blood products (for any reason whatsoever) due to the increased possibility of needing a blood transfusion, and I council any patient considering bilateral TKR that there is a very good chance (better than 70 percent) that they will require such a transfusion.

Two Hips or One?

Before we conclude this chapter, you'll notice that there is no chapter in this handbook entitled "Two Hips or One?" The reason for this is simple, I do not believe that any patient should consider having both hips replaced at once. A hip replacement is a bigger operation than knee replacement. The hip joints are deeper than your knee joints and therefore the surgery is more invasive, with more tissue dissection, and more blood loss during the operation. In the knee, we have the luxury of using tourniquets to limit blood loss to almost nothing during the surgery (which we cannot use in hip replacement surgery). There are, however, good orthopedic surgeons who would disagree with me on this matter. If that is your strong preference, I recommend researching which surgeons in your area perform bilateral hip replacements on a regular basis, and schedule a visit to discuss your individual situation.

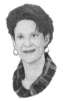 **Campone's Comment:** While I defer to Dr. Hugate's recognition that some surgeons may be willing to undertake bilateral hip replacement, my own experience suggests that there are significant reasons for not doing so beyond purely medical considerations. The surgery is, as noted here, quite extensive and requires

considerable time and energy for following through on all that is required in the recovery and healing processes, as I speak about in *Chapter 6, Journey Through Two Hip Replacements*. There is a considerable period of downtime in recovery from the trauma of the surgical procedure and, for me at least, to fully recover from the effects of anesthesia. Furthermore, there are significant limitations on movement until the joint is well along in the recovery process, so ordinary movements such as walking are very slow and deliberate and, for a time, may require the use of an assistive device. Other ordinary movements such as bending are severely restricted for a period of time as well.

An important aspect of recovery entails regaining a sense of competency. Having one functioning joint gave me a point of reference for what was still working instead of a sense of helplessness and pervasiveness about what was wounded. I could comfort myself by flexing what I could while regaining that ability with the joint I couldn't flex. Being able to start walking with at least one working hip was essential to my maintaining a sense of control. ~*~

This is a lot of information, but I've tried to boil it down and clarify it for you. Keep all of these points in mind as you ask yourself these extremely important questions, and you should be able to make an educated and well-considered decision.

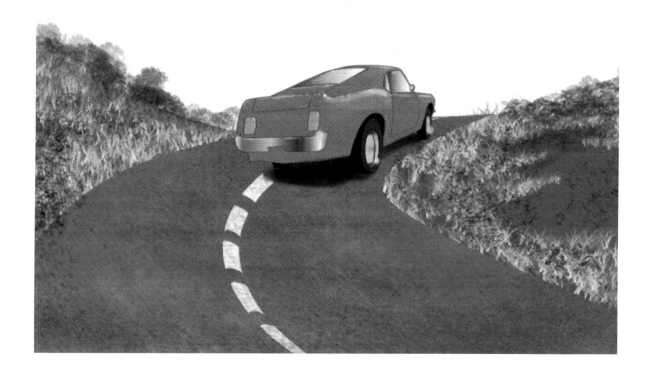

Journey Through 2 Hip Replacements

AHEAD

Journey Through Two Hip Replacements

CHAPTER 6

by Francine Campone

A few years before my 2005 move to Denver, Colorado, I started to get messages from my left hip. Walking—ouch! Getting up from a chair—ouch! Dancing—ouch, ouch! At the time, I decided to ignore these, as I would with any junk mail. Over about six months, however, the messages became more insistent and persistent, and I finally decided to listen. Since I lived in a small city at the time, with one major hospital, I asked a friend—a former nurse and the wife of an anesthesiologist at the hospital—for a recommendation. Thinking what I had was a pulled muscle, I showed up for the appointment, walked when asked to walk, stood when asked to stand, and held still for a series of X-rays. When the doctor showed me a picture of a raggedy-ended joint and used the "A" word (arthritis), it didn't quite register.

The doctor assured me that the arthritis was not yet sufficiently advanced to consider hip replacement and, anyway, he told me I was too young to consider the surgery as the replacement would be expected to last only about fifteen plus years and then I would need another. While it was something of a relief to hear that I was too young for something, I wasn't quite convinced that he was right about the whole thing. He recommended that I do some non-impact exercises (such as cycling or swimming) and invited me back when I felt the time was right.

Hugate's Comment: Hip pain can sometimes be a bit tricky to figure out because there are so many different causes. Hip pain from arthritis usually causes pain in the groin area of the hip. It's usually worse with activity, especially rotation of the hip or while lifting the leg. Pain on the outer part of the hip can also be from arthritis, but other causes would include bursitis or even pinched nerves in the back sending pain into the hip area. Francine describes the progression of her pain eloquently. Pain levels tend to start out annoying and progress

71

to debilitating over the course of a few years in those with arthritis. A quick visit to the doctor for an examination and X-ray will show defini- tively if arthritis is the culprit. ~*~

When people are confronted with a significant and sudden loss, they tend to follow a pattern of grieving: denial, anger, and bargaining usually all precede acceptance. While I didn't realize it at the time, I had started down that road, albeit getting stuck for a while in denial. Arthritis, in my mental model of the world, was an *old person's disease* and at just past fifty years of age, I was not an *old person*! Thinking about it made me cranky. Then I tried bargaining. While I am not given to following orders, I took up the exercise suggestion and bought myself an excellent stationary-bike which I alternated with exercise classes at the new city pool. Perhaps the heavy course of fish oil (recommended by a friend in New York who was fighting the same battle) helped me stay afloat. Surely, I thought, exercising would keep this thing at bay. While the twinges and occasional pain did not go away, the situation was bearable enough that I continued on that course for about three years. During that time, I felt depressed and, ultimately, resigned to cranking around with pain (because pain makes me cranky and I suspect it does for you too).

After my husband, Ed, and I moved to Denver, I was inspired by the healthy Colorado lifestyle and a serious warning from my family physician about the need to lose at least fifty pounds. While the doctor had prescribed an anti-inflammatory medication for me to manage my now-increasing hip pain, he also warned of the possible long-term side effects. Another set of X-rays showed that the joint degeneration had significantly increased and that the cartilage in both hips was starting to wear down to the bone. The doctor and my husband had both suggested that my excess weight might be aggravating the problem, but denial in that area prevailed for a long time too.

There is another model called "stages of readiness for change" (derived from studies of people trying to change addictive behaviors such as smoking and drinking). Denial is the first stage of this journey as well, a resistance to any suggestion that a change is needed. Once the message about a need for change gets through, the next stage is contemplation. I did quite a bit of thinking about losing weight, made some half-hearted efforts at a diet and played around the edges of making a real effort to do what I knew deep in my unconscious needed to be done. But everyone has a breaking point when the discomfort of the present situation outweighs the possible challenges posed by actually committing to make behavioral changes. In my case, the now relentless hip pain, coupled with the medical problems that may accompany being overweight, eventually motivated me to change from thinking about to doing. I joined an effective weight loss program and stuck with it faithfully, documenting everything I ate, measuring and weighing my food, and intentionally transferring mental energy from resistance to commitment. Over the course of a year and a half, I dropped a total of sixty-five pounds. This proved to be highly beneficial in reducing the risks in the surgery, and is likely to have contributed to a smoother recovery in the long run.

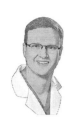 **Hugate's Comment:** *Kudos to Francine for being able to pull off that amount of weight loss. We often recommend weight loss as a strategy to help alleviate pressure on the joints, but it is much easier said than done. Of course, there are secondary benefits to overall health as well with weight loss. There is no doubt that by committing to that level of weight loss, Francine reduced the stress on her arthritic joints. Further, when it came time to replace those joints, her risk for complications was significantly reduced as well. ~*~*

While my slimmer self felt better physically, mentally, and emotionally, any movements that might be in the neighborhood of exercise, including walking and hiking, remained painful. My trusted family practitioner referred me to an orthopedist who took new X-rays and did a thorough assessment of various dimensions of the experience, including pain level. He indicated that at that point, both hips were suitable for replacement surgery but that I need not proceed until I felt my quality of life had been negatively impacted enough to undertake the surgery. We also discussed the rehabilitation after surgery and he admonished me to not proceed until I was committed to seeing things through completely.

That took about a year—mostly because I'm very stubborn. But when I experienced serious pain while walking, standing, lying down, and sitting... well, I didn't have much choice. Hip pain interfered with sleeping soundly, which in turn had a domino effect on daily activities. Also, I was tired of carrying a walking stick, something I had taken up to relieve the pressure on my joints during even ordinary activities. And I was still cranky! Chronic pain is a great contributor to distorting even a usually calm and generally content disposition, as my husband and colleagues can attest. The impact of the condition rippled well beyond me, affecting loved ones in my immediate circle. Ed and I no longer enjoyed many shared activities, both pleasurable—like walks in the Denver Botanic Gardens—and ordinary—like grocery shopping. Detrimental fallout, both physical and emotional, reached a critical tipping point and I was ready to do whatever it took to make the pain stop.

So Ed and I went back to my surgeon and made the date. My doctor is a hip-and-knee replacement specialist and had extensive experience with replacing these joints. One thing I especially liked is that he had a whole team and one of his prerequisites for surgery was attending a two-hour workshop with his other patients about to get joint replacements. In that session, we met the team, including the physical and occupational therapists who would work with us post-surgery, and the nurse liaison from the hospital. The doctor's assistant gave a full overview of what to expect on the day of surgery and during the recovery period, both in the hospital and at home. We learned the various precautions and limitations on movement during the approximately three-month period when muscles were regaining elasticity. We were introduced to the various assistive devices available and recommended. Then we passed around a joint implant: titanium, modular, and much smaller and lighter than I had expected. The session ended with application forms for temporary parking permits so I could use handicapped spots.

It also ended with a sigh of relief. Knowing what to expect is a great antidote to fear. Studies in neuroscience show that the brain has a primal, emotional part and a more logical, rational part. Like most human beings, my most primal emotions, when heightened, tend to overwhelm the voices of reason in my brain. But I'm a thoughtful person by nature, so for me, getting information helps the logical part of my brain "talk back" to the emotional part in these situations and helps balance feelings with rational thought. That's why this information session had a calming effect on me.

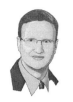 **Hugate's Comment:** This is a wonderful service offered by most hospitals where joint replacements are performed: the "joint replacement class." Here you can meet the providers, talk about the process, and ask questions. It takes a great deal of the anxiety out of the event. Most often, representatives from nursing, physical therapy, occupational therapy, and sometimes the operating room may be present at the class. The goal is to inform you preemptively about what you will go through (and what will be required of you) during the joint replacement journey. I strongly encourage you to seek out and attend such a class if your hospital offers it. ~*~

Nonetheless, as the date approached I felt butterflies. I'm a long-time meditation practitioner and a part of me knew that the feelings were natural and were just feelings, waves of experience that come and go. I did my best to keep busy, which wasn't hard given that there was a pile of work to complete before the *big day*. As a self-employed executive coach and a faculty member who teaches in a virtual classroom, I had the luxury of setting my own schedule for the event and planning downtime in the aftermath.

With my first hip replacement in 2008, I wasn't sure what to expect but—overconfident as ever—I figured that two weeks would be enough for me to at least be up to talking on the phone and working at my laptop, albeit keeping a light schedule.

I can't say I remember much about the surgery, except that I went onto the operating table with pain and woke up much later feeling... okay. Discomfort, yes, but the burning sensation I had learned to live with was gone. Of course, I was numbed somewhat from the anesthesia. The good side to this was that when the physical therapist came in later that day and invited me to get out of bed and make my way over to the chair, I hazily consented and perhaps was even cheerful about it. In the days that followed, I created a routine of breakfast, wash up, morning physical and occupational therapy, lunch, afternoon therapy, dinner. This experience and the routine that followed when I went home set a new pattern that I learned to put to good use in the years that followed.

The first few days home were, as predicted, disorienting. I found myself sleeping most of the day; the physician's team had stressed that it was important to do this. As someone who is usually active and engaged, I found it difficult at first to give myself permission to just sleep and to not need to do anything particularly productive when awake. Audio books became my best friends during this period. Ed had been prepared as much as I had, so he was able to strike just the right balance between loving caretaking and encouragement to engage in those actions that would promote my recovery. This included sleeping as much as necessary, eating well, and doing the daily, physical therapy routines I had been prescribed. Ed got me up and walking every day. The first few days, it was a slow shuffle with the walker around the corridor of our apartment building, circling the elevator bank once, then going around twice and continuing until—after a few days—I was bored to tears and ready for new scenery. I rattled my way with the walker from the bedroom to the living room and stood at the open balcony door. Every morning when I woke up, I left my loving taskmaster sleeping and went into the living room to do the first of three daily sets of prescribed stretches. It was not exactly fun but every inch further that I could move the reconstructed hip was proof I was going to be fine.

Indoor shuffling around soon gave way to getting back to the great outdoors. I studied the photos in the handbook of how to go up and down stairs in preparation for navigating the three steps in the building entryway. In truth, we do have a very nice ramp but it's just my nature to push the boundaries, and do what I can on my own behalf before I ask someone else to do for me. Many friends offered to take me out for an airing and relieve Ed and we happily accepted. At first, my outing consisted of a walk up and down the block. Then I was able to go around the block. Finally, walking the three blocks from our home to the entrance of the Denver Botanic Gardens was cause for celebration. I set that as a benchmark because I so enjoy the Gardens and find it a restoring and energizing place to spend time.

Because the surgery had taken place the first week of October, I had a few months of outdoor walking before winter weather slowed that process down. I became very cautious about icy sidewalks, and I'm still tentative walking far in inclement weather.

Within a few weeks of starting the outdoor program, I was able to graduate from using a walker to a cane. Perhaps I expedited this a bit, as I found that nothing ages a woman more than using a walker, and frankly, my vanity still wasn't ready to give up that battle. Shortly thereafter, I traded in my conventional hook-top cane for a lightweight hiking pole, which felt somehow jauntier. I checked in regularly with the doctor and kept up my morning stretching, doing the full routine while the coffee brewed. The swelling that distorted the left side of my body slowly went down and the more colorful skin tones (black, blue, purple, yellow, and other shades) eventually faded to a normal pink.

Once I was back to full speed, I felt reborn! Getting the left hip replaced eliminated the chronic pain, self-consciousness, and *dis-ease* that had come to take over my mental and physical life. It was only with that freedom that I realized how constricted my life had become. Along with this recognition came an appreciation for the opportunities inherent in this liberation. One of these opportunities lay in the morning routine I established of exercising while the coffee brews. Physical exercise has never been high on my "A-list" of activities, although I love to dance, enjoy a moderate hike with Ed, and can get myself onto my exercise bike on occasion. Since I had a new routine, I decided to gradually replace the outmoded elements of the physical therapy regimen with other exercises. So I began (with the go-ahead from the doctor) to add in some gentle yoga stretches. The doctor's guidance was good common sense: if it doesn't feel right, don't do it. The new practice of a morning exercise routine became an integral part of my daily life and I have maintained that practice to this day.

A parallel opportunity in this newly regained life was found in a reconnection between body and mind. I am by nature, inclination, and training a somewhat sedentary and thinking sort of person. Much of the time, my attention is focused on what's going on in the head rather than how the head and body are synchronizing with each other. The body-mind connection comes to the fore during periods of physical stress when the body simply shouts for and gains attention. In my case, the bad hip brought my attention to other places in my life that were similarly hobbled by thoughts, feelings, and choices. I noticed dimensions of lifestyle where I felt I was no longer hitting my stride, taking big enough steps, or covering new ground. I recognized that I could use this newly regained awareness to cultivate attunement to how states of mind affect the physical self and vice-versa. The recovery period also offered a place for recalibrating work-life balance. In day-to-day life, I began to pay attention to spine alignment when sitting, to use my core muscles more when walking and to make it a point to get up and move periodically throughout a workday at the computer. The positive impact on my mental state was undeniable.

Inevitably, my right hip got jealous of the flexibility and sense of well-being in the left and started to send similar signals demanding a change! As with the first hip, occasional discomfort became pain, occasional pain became steady pain, and there was a significant impairment in day-to-day functioning. When I asked my doctor when I'd be ready for the second operation, he replied, "You will know." A key lesson from the first replacement was a determination to not wait as long the second time around. Nonetheless, work commitments prevented me from finding a "good time"—thinking not so much about the surgery and hospital time as the downtime I could expect afterward.

Recovery from hip replacement is a slow process. In particular, as I was reminded over and over again, hip replacement surgery is a significant trauma to the body and requires considerable rest in order to allow the body to repair itself. All my life, I have required only a moderate amount of sleep: 6-1/2 hours a night serves me perfectly well. In the hospital, the night nurse (who agreed to bring me coffee in the mornings to temper the gruesomely early wake-up), was emphatic about taking the prescribed painkillers and sleeping pills, even though I didn't feel the need. When I returned home after the first surgery, I found myself sleeping nine hours a night and taking two to three naps a day (without the support of the prescribed pain medications). The second time around, I did allow myself a longer period of downtime without appointments and notified clients and university staff I'd be out of commission for a month. This gave me permission to genuinely relax and sleep without a mental to-do list running through my head during the day. As it turned out, while I did still sleep long nights and need a nap during the day, recovery from the second surgery proceeded much more quickly and with less discomfort.

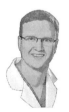

Hugate's Comment: The increased amount of sleep that Francine describes here is perfectly normal after joint replacement surgery and can be due to a number of factors. First of all, you've just been injured (in a controlled fashion) by your surgery, so your body goes into a catabolic state in which it requires more rest and more calories to function and repair itself. In addition, pain medications can cause you to be drowsy.

As for returning to work: I generally advise my patients to take six weeks off from work if they're in a sedentary profession (a profession that does not involve significant lifting, climbing, crawling, jumping, pushing, pulling, and so on). If your job is more labor intensive, then I would recommend planning on three months out of work. Patients will often be able to return to work sooner, but if you set the expectation at six weeks and come back sooner, you are perceived as a dedicated worker who returned to work "ahead of schedule." On the other hand, if you tell your boss you'll *be out for a month, and instead it takes you six weeks to recover, you'll be perceived as failing to return to work on schedule. This is a subtle point, but one worth making. These timelines also allow you to rest mentally and physically, rather than rushing to get back into stressful situations. Do yourself a favor and take the time you need to recover fully. ~*~*

My surgeon had suggested that this is often the case. In part, it may be that the mind knows what to expect, and that knowledge, combined with a successful first outcome, can have a significant impact on reducing fear. Also, in the two years between my first and second replacement surgeries, the joint replacement implant became smaller and lighter, downsizing some aspects of the surgical procedure. Further, the success of the first THR planted an expectation of similar success for the second. Recent studies in neuroscience and positive psychology underscore the role of expectations and mental models in framing experiences. Once again, the body-mind link was reinforced through measuring the relative speed of recovery from the second with the successful results of the first. As I had retained the habit of morning stretching and exercise, it was easy to replace my yoga routine with the prescribed physical therapy. The second surgery took place in June of 2010, which made it much easier to start the outdoor walking regimen, as the sidewalks were dry and the weather inviting. Expectation of a positive outcome for my efforts provided a strong motivator to continue following the prescribed routine.

This entire journey has itself been a motivator. For me, those first simple messages from my left hip turned into an ongoing internal dialogue about body and mind, life choices, relationships, commitments, and change. It is a conversation that no one can avoid, especially those of us in what some psychologists refer to as "The Third Age" (the period, post-middle age, when individuals have opportunities for creative reinvention and application of the wisdom, skills, and resources acquired in the first half of life). While major surgery is not an experience that one seeks, when the need for such surgery arises, it offers a path to reinventing oneself physically, mentally, and spiritually. If your hips are calling, listen, and choose your answer carefully.

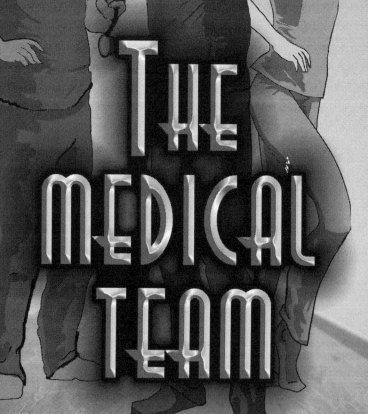

Your Medical Team

by Dr. Hugate

Caring for patients is a team event. Make no mistake, the surgeon is the captain of that team, but without all the members of the team doing their jobs well, there will not be a good outcome. I could write an entire book on the dedicated individuals who contribute to your success when you decide to have surgery. Some of them you see, and some of them you don't. From the hospital administration insuring that we have all the latest and best equipment, to the hospital staff who sterilize the surgical instruments and clean the operating rooms (ORs) to lessen your risk of infection, we're all working toward one goal: to perform your surgery in a safe and efficient manner and get you back to your life—without the pain! The purpose of this chapter is to introduce you to a *few* of the key team members whom you will interact with during your joint replacement journey and to give you an idea of what each of their roles is, both in the hospital and out.

Primary Care Provider (PCP)

Your medical team starts with your *Primary Care Provider* (PCP). PCPs continually amaze me with the breadth of their knowledge. They're asked to be orthopedic specialists one minute, and the very next minute may have a dermatological or gynecological issue to attend to. They're able to "swap hats" as easily as you or I change our socks. A good PCP is a life-long friend who knows your medical history better than anyone. She can medically manage a myriad of complex chronic conditions. If your hips or knees are bothering you, the best place to get an initial evaluation is your PCP. It's likely that she will help initially recognize—and diagnose—that you have arthritis and make the appropriate referral to consult with an orthopedic surgeon when the time is right.

Office Staff

Your surgeon's team becomes involved as soon as you make the phone call to their office. The front office staff manages the phones, receiving new patient requests and sets up your appointments for you. A good office staff can help comfort you with their words and get you in to see the doctor in a timely manner to discuss your problems. Office staffers have a number of responsibilities, including making appointments, managing medical records, performing X-rays, insurance verification, billing, scheduling surgery, and triaging patient's phone calls.

Most offices assign a *medical assistant* (MA) to each physician. The MA is the office staff member who is the "right hand" of the doctor and the treatment team. The MA is often the one who greets you at the door with a smile when it's time to see the surgeon and walks you back to your examination room. He may get your vital signs and even get a brief history about your symptoms before any of your treatment team sees you. He will often be the one to help coordinate any records that need to be assembled, including lab results, doctors' reports, and X-rays. The MA is also the staff member who first accepts your phone call if you have treatment questions, and he will either answer your questions or pass them along to the appropriate treatment team member.

The individual in charge of the office staff is the *office manager*. Her job is to keep the office staff running smoothly and to assure the patients are happy and well taken care of. If you have any issues you're not happy about regarding office operations, the office manager is the person to ask for.

Treatment Team:

Physician Extenders

Now for the treatment team: The treatment team generally consists of your doctor and, quite often, either a nurse or a "physician extender." We've already discussed the surgeon's role in your care, so let's focus here on the role of the physician extender. Physician extenders are a group of professionals who are highly trained and very good at what they do. Their job is to be the second set of eyes and ears for your surgeon and support the process of patient care every step of the way—essentially *extending* the ability of the physician to care for all of his patients more efficiently. They see patients in the clinic, after surgery in the hospital, and may even assist the surgeon during surgery. Their titles are either *physician assistant* (PA), or sometimes *nurse practitioner* (NP). These professionals undergo extensive medical training to gain the title of PA or NP and then go on to gain valuable experience working in their particular field. They are licensed in their fields and credentialed by the hospital. They usually practice under the direct supervision of a physician (although in some states they can practice independently). Physician extenders work closely with their doctor, and the good ones know exactly how their physician thinks and what that physician would want or do in almost any clinical scenario.

Not all surgeons have physician extenders, but if your surgeon does, there's a good chance that you may visit him before you see the surgeon. His job during your initial visit is to go through your medical and surgical history and organize the information for presentation to your surgeon. This allows your surgeon to get a concise picture of the issues concerning your case and hone right in on those issues. Essentially the physician extender allows the surgeon to spend more time with you face-to-face and not thumbing through the chart looking up details. The physician extender will also likely be responsible for taking medical questions by phone (after the MA has triaged), and contacting you with solutions to those problems after discussion with your surgeon; thus, he is another very important part of your team.

Surgical Team

Next let's talk about the *anesthesiologist*. An anesthesiologist is a physician who specializes in keeping you safe and comfortable during surgery and sometimes even helps with pain control after surgery through various methods. This can mean anything from going completely to sleep (general anesthesia) to having some sort of nerve block which numbs a specific area of your body long enough for the surgeon to complete the procedure. Anesthesiologists are experts in pharmacology and physiology and have a number of "tricks" in their bag to get you in and out of surgery safely and comfortably. The purpose of having an anesthesiologist present is to have one highly skilled set of dedicated eyes and ears on you at all times while the surgeon performs the procedure. This allows your surgeon to focus on his technically demanding task with the comfort of knowing that you (the patient) are being watched closely by another provider throughout. ***Chapter 9, Anesthesia Options in Joint Replacement Surgery*** is dedicated to all of the anesthesia options, so I won't belabor the point now. Suffice it to say that the anesthesiologist is a key member of the surgical team who is primarily responsible for your health and well-being during the course of the procedure.

The *surgical assistant* (SA) and *scrub tech* are two other important team members at work during your surgery. You may or may not have a chance to formally meet them before the procedure. SAs and scrub techs are trained, licensed providers in their respective fields and credentialed by the hospital. Their main job is to help the surgeon perform the procedure safely and efficiently. Routine surgical procedures, such as hip or knee replacements, are really an orchestrated series of events occurring in a particular sequence—much like a concert. (We'll describe this concert in much greater detail in **Chapter 11, The Operations**.) The SA is primarily responsible for retracting tissue and positioning the leg so that the surgeon can visualize and access the structures necessary to perform the operation safely. The SA or PA may also help suture the wound closed at the end of the procedure. The scrub tech is mainly responsible for organizing and delivering the surgical instruments and implants to the surgeon. A good surgical team (surgeon, surgical assistant, scrub tech) will often go through a procedure such as joint replacement without saying much to one another at all. This is because each knows the next step and they move forward "automatically" in concert. The scrub tech and SA spend the entire time in the operating room closely anticipating the surgeon's next move and working to make the procedure as smooth and seamless as possible. This, in turn, reduces the time required to perform the operation, which reduces the risk of complications, such as issues associated with anesthesia or risk of infection.

Nurses

Nurses are the life-blood of any hospital. You'll meet a nurse as soon as you hit the doors of the admitting area and one will very likely walk you down to your car on the day of your discharge. There are nurses in the preoperative area, in the OR during surgery, in the recovery room, and on the orthopedics floor where you're taken for the few days after surgery. From beginning to end of your stay at the hospital, nurses will be greeting you, assessing you, administering medications, and generally *taking care* of you. A good nurse will be nurturing and pleasant but firm when necessary. They're innately able to comfort patients and family members. Their actions and judgments during your stay will have the most significant impact on your safety and comfort. While the surgeon will see you once a day when in the hospital, a nurse will be assigned to you around the clock at all times. They typically work eight-hour shifts during the week, so they will rotate your care as the day passes. The nurses' responsibilities are broad. They will collect vital signs at regular intervals and record them on your chart. Pain, mental status, nerve function, and pulse (heart rate) are included in your vital sign assessment as well. (We speak a great deal more about this in *Chapter 13, The Hospital Stay*.) Your nurses will administer medications according to a set of postoperative orders. They'll arrange for labs to be drawn according to the doctor's orders, and if anything of concern comes up, they're able to contact the treatment team at any time and manage the situation as necessary. Your nurses are your best friends and strongest allies in the days following surgery.

The Hospitalist

You may also have a second physician on your care team while in the hospital. "Hospitalists" are medical doctors (usually internal medicine specialists) who specialize in taking care of patients admitted to the hospital. On some occasions, your PCP may fulfill this role, but more commonly after surgery, if you have any medical issues, the hospitalist will manage them while you're in the hospital. She will gather your medical information, family history, previous labs and tests, and so on, and work alongside your surgeon. On occasion, if there are a number of complex medical issues, your surgeon may refer you to visit the hospitalist before the day of surgery so the two of you can become acquainted. You'll typically meet the hospitalist fairly soon after your surgery, and she will see you daily or more frequently if needed. Most hospitals have a hospitalist on duty twenty-four hours a day (they also rotate in shifts). This means that you'll have a physician on direct standby around the clock should any issues arise. While the surgeon manages routine postoperative issues and postoperative pain control, the hospitalists may, for example, manage your insulin dose (if you're diabetic), or your blood pressure pills (if you have high blood pressure). A good hospitalist works and communicates with your surgeon closely to greatly increase your odds for a good outcome.

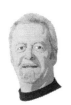 **Holland's Comment:** *In addition, during the pre-operative hiatus, your surgeon will ensure that any other "conditional specialists" whose care you're under (such as a heart specialist) also examine you and give their direct, written authorization affirming you're in good enough health to proceed. If you're under the care of any other specialists your PCP might be unaware of (and this can easily be the case due to the new insurance rules), talk about them with your surgeon and let the other specialists know what your plans are too.* ~*~

Therapists (PT and OT)

You will also meet a physical therapist (PT) while you are in the hospital. (In *Chapter 14, Physical Therapy for Hip and Knee Replacement Surgery*, we describe in detail the role of this important provider in your recovery.) Most surgeons have you start physical therapy soon after surgery. Your surgeon writes orders which describe how much weight you're allowed to put on the leg and how much you should move the joint. The PT takes the ball and runs from there. You'll likely have physical therapy at least twice a day while in the hospital. A good PT is compassionate but firm. If you have joint replacement and then make it your goal thereafter to keep your joint in a comfortable position, your outcome may not be the best. It's the job of the PT to get you outside your comfort zone and move the joint early and often so this doesn't happen.

Once you leave the hospital, you'll be referred to an outpatient physical therapist in the community. It is this therapist who will spend more time with you than any other health professional during the initial six weeks after surgery. You'll see your PT as much as three times a week for six to eight weeks and even more if your motion doesn't progress according to schedule. You'll grow to have a love-hate relationship with your physical therapist, but always remember that his primary goal is to help you restore your function!

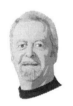 **Holland's Comment:** Also, you'll be meeting an Occupational Therapist (OT) whose specialty is helping you learn to reestablish your function and independence after surgery. He does this by helping you perform your so-called: Activities of Daily Living (ADLs)—like putting on your socks, getting in and out of your car, picking things up when you can't bend over, bathing and going to the bathroom using a walker, crutches, or cane—when needed. In addition, both your OT and PT are also closely involved in evaluating whether you're able (and ready) to be released from the hospital after surgery. We'll cover this in much greater detail in *Chapter 13, The Hospital Stay.* However, part of your OT's job both at home and in the hospital is to help you learn to perform the practical tasks of living better, safer and easier. Their help in teaching you how to paddle your boat down the river of life is an essential part of your journey through joint replacement.

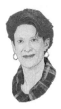

Campone's Comment: In addition to the team members mentioned by Dr. Hugate, my THR team included a hospital liaison who was available to help out with any questions or issues specifically related to my hospital stay. The hospital liaison was also helpful in directing us to the appropriate office for billing and insurance issues and in managing the process of acquiring assistive devices prior to my discharge after surgery. ~*~

   This chapter mentions a few of the key professionals you'll meet during the process of joint replacement surgery. There are more, to be sure, and I could go on for pages, but we've covered the most visible players on the team—the ones you're most likely to interact with. Remember that what we do on a routine basis may not be routine to you, so never hesitate to ask any professional on your team about his or her role in your care. Also, keep in mind that while you're the patient and you're supposed to cooperate in helping us help you, you're also the *customer,* and as such, you have the ultimate say over what goes on.

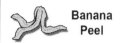 **Banana Peel**
 Throw Rug
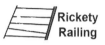 **Rickety Railing**
 Electrical Cording
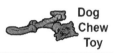 **Dog Chew Toy**

Find the Tripping Hazards Above in the Picture Below

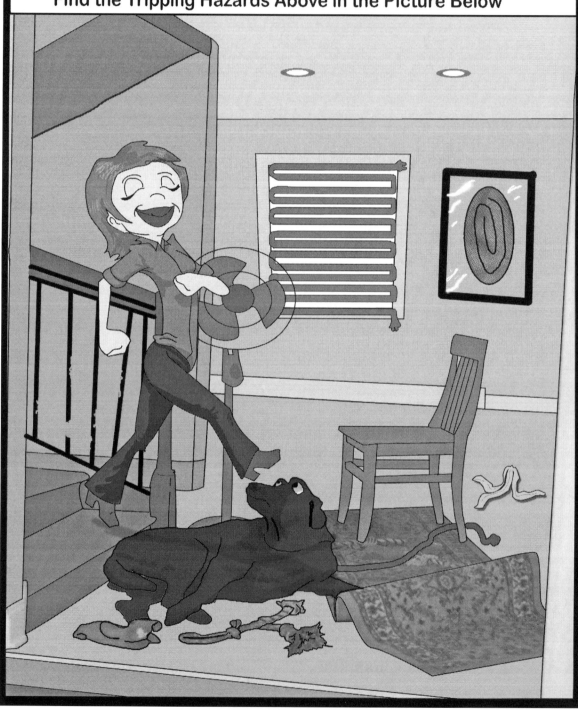

Preparing Your Home

CHAPTER 8

by Mr. Holland

By now we've shared a great deal of information about getting this journey underway. If you've decided to proceed with joint replacement surgery, you'll need to spend some time preparing your home (to the best of your ability and finances). In every case of the journey through joint replacement, one of the greatest fears people have, and one of the greatest risks to the new surgery itself, is "falling". So we'll begin by discussing this important topic.

Obviously, the world presents us with opportunities to fall all the time, so we'll limit our discussion here to some of the issues that may be risk factors in your home. Simply put, to adequately prepare your home, you'll want to eliminate as many risks for falling as you can. In truth, this subject could warrant an entire handbook in itself. We'll focus on the major points of concern and identify resources for you to research further should you so desire. I've included some photos which can act as guidelines, but—in general—if you find yourself reaching out to hold on to a corner for balance, grabbing the doorways as you pass through, or find yourself hugging the wall for safety, this is an area of concern for falling. Falls occur most frequently in the kitchen, bathroom, and stairs, so you should focus on these areas especially.

Hugate's Comment: You'll recall from Francine's writing in Chapter 6, Journey Through Two Hip Replacements, that while having your joint replaced won't make you any older, you will move very gingerly (like a very old person) early in the rehabilitation process while at home. Falls can be problematic and may even set your recovery back.

You need to be thinking about managing this risk in a preventative manner both before and after surgery. Generally speaking, those people who fit the following descriptions—before surgery—are at the greatest risk for injury from a fall at home:

- Those who used a walker or crutches before surgery
- Having a history of balance problems or falling
- Obese people
- Age greater than 65 years
- Those who live alone
- People with osteoporosis (thin bones)

Patients in these groups are at higher risk for injury from falling and should consider making extra home preparations before undergoing joint replacement. If you fit into any of these categories, read this chapter carefully and strongly consider making any modifications we've recommended.
~*~

Tripping Hazards

There are more common tripping hazards in the home than you may realize. Throw rugs are notorious for causing trip-and-fall events. As such, before joint replacement these should be removed altogether. The kind without a non-slip backing simply don't provide a stable base to walk on—no matter what type of hard-surface, or carpeted floor, they're on. Furthermore, even if they do have a non-slip backing, they often bunch up, and even a slight irregularity can trip you. The takeaway here is that no matter the type or location, throw rugs can cause an unexpected trip-and-fall event. Moreover, any minor irregularities in your floors: uneven (or broken) floor boards, loose tiles, damaged thresholds, and so on, should be repaired to reduce the risk from these unperceived hazards. Extension cords and lamp cords are a notorious source of falls—especially when laid across common walking pathways. In addition, pet toys, pet food bowls, pet beds, etc., should all be placed in an area where they aren't in your normal, household traffic patterns.

There are areas in your home without tripping hazards, per se, which still present a risk for falling. These are generally areas which have a constrained walking space, such as: stairwells, bathrooms, bedrooms and kitchens. These areas often have very hard objects or hard surfaces, such as: tile (or wood) floors, furniture, kitchen appliances, sinks, toilets, bathtubs, steps, etc., all of which can magnify potential injury from a fall. If you have stairs in your home—and there's any doubt whatsoever as to their integrity—have them inspected (especially the handrails), and make repairs if needed. You'll be using your handrails to support yourself a great deal more than you normally would—meaning they must be up to the task. Some stairs have rug-runners, stair tread covers, etc. (See Figure 8.2) which must be securely fastened down or removed.

Obviously , you must also be able to see where you're walking. The most common walking paths within a home are hallways to and from: the bedrooms, bathrooms, living areas, and kitchen. All common pathways in the home, including walking areas around furniture, must be well-lit both day and night—especially the first few weeks after surgery. Strategic placement of night-lights will often suffice. These days some very pretty, glow-plate, plug-in luminaires (that use almost no energy) are readily available. Having your walking areas well illuminated will seriously improve your ability to navigate through your house safely. To sum up this section of our handbook:

If you identify an area of your home that may be problematic after joint replacement—it should be addressed proactively.

Arranging Your Home During Recovery

You can also reduce the risk for falling by reducing the amount of walking you need to do. By this we mean arranging your home in such a way that you don't need to go far to get what you need. Before joint replacement, you should set your home up so you can live on the main floor for the first couple of weeks after surgery. Ideally your bedroom, bathroom, and kitchen should all be on the same floor (to reduce the need for using stairs). Make sure that whatever area you set up for your temporary quarters has safe and easy egress from the house in case of emergency.

Another trick to reduce the amount of walking you need to do is to take care of any routine household chores before you going for surgery. For example, prepare some frozen meals which can be warmed in a microwave oven—thus saving you the chore of cooking right after surgery. Wash all your laundry before going to the hospital so you don't have to bother with this for the first couple of weeks back at home. Make sure your pantry and refrigerator are well stocked so you're not forced to go out and pick up food, and speak with your local grocer to see if they deliver—find one that will. Make sure all of your prescription medications are refilled (a thirty-day supply is ideal), so you don't have to make any unexpected trips to the pharmacy either. This should include a supply of over-the-counter, stool softeners for use while on pain medications after surgery, as pain medications can cause constipation. Pet care, lawn care, snow and trash removal should all be prearranged as well. The fewer of these mundane chores you have on your plate after joint replacement, the less your risk of falling.

One of the most comprehensive resource for guidelines on preparing your home for safety (no matter where you are in the world) is the official, U.S. government website for the Americans with Disabilities Act (ADA) and there are many other resources at your local library. Of course, we (as joint replacement patients) aren't government agencies or public venues trying accomplish ADA compliance, our objective is—quite simply—is to have a safe and uneventful recovery. Here are the web addresses to the U.S. government websites and files which outline the ADA recommendations:

www.ada.gov/

www.ada.gov/regs2010/2010ADAStandards/2010ADAStandards.pdf

What if You Do Fall?

OK—so what if, despite all of these precautions, you take a fall? What then? We recommend a few measures. First, keep a charged cellular phone with you at all times with pre-programmed phone numbers for neighbors, friends, family, and emergency services. If you have a spouse (significant other, or at-home caregiver), make sure he or she keeps their own phone charged up and turned on just in case you need help, or have fallen and can't get up.

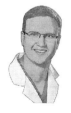 **Hugate's Comment:** Also think about getting a medical alert bracelet if you have any major medical problems. This will alert anyone who may come to help as to what medical problems you have. There are also services in many communities that provide a "notification locket." This is basically a push-button device you can put around your neck that alerts a help center when pushed. When alerted, the help center will call to verify if you're OK; if you can't answer, they will send help. I also recommend that if you live alone, arrange for someone to visit you at least twice a day and check on you for the first three weeks after surgery at the very minimum. ~*~

Special Hip Replacement Considerations

If you have undergone hip replacement surgery you should not bend your hip beyond 90 degrees when sitting down, getting to your feet, or bending over. Our handbook describes the Hip Precautions in much greater detail in **Chapter 14, Physical Therapy for Hip and Knee Replacement**. One situation in which this occurs is that of sitting in a low chair that makes your knees end up higher than your hips (See Figure 8.1). Chairs such as the one depicted below—in the photo of me on the right—put you at risk for dislocation after hip replacement surgery.

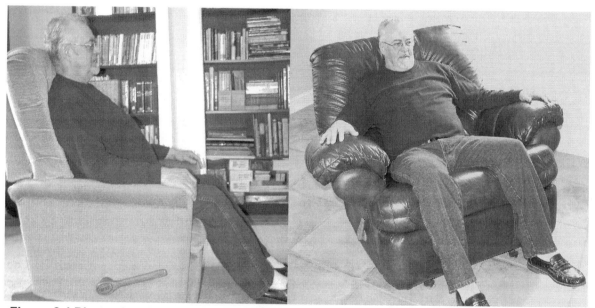

Figure 8.1 Photo showing two chairs; on the left the chair is high enough (knees are not above hips), and on the right, the chair is too low (knees are above hips)

Hugate's comment: Robert is absolutely right here. No matter if it's your "favorite chair" or not, if you're having a hip replacement, low chairs must go! And don't be fooled by that big fluffy chair, it may look like a high-enough seat, but once you sit on it—and sink into it—it's now a low chair, especially (as Robert points out) when trying to get up. Here's a test you can try before going in for hip surgery: fully seat yourself in the chair and if your knees are higher off the ground than your hips, or if you bend excessively getting up, it's a 'low chair' and you shouldn't use it. ~*~

Examples Concerning Your Home:

Stairwells and Floor Clutter:

—> <u>Eliminate trip-and-fall hazards.</u> Fasten stair runners in place and especially remove loose, throw rugs nearby stair landings.

Depending on your individual circumstances, you may be using a cane, a set of crutches, or even a walker for a few weeks (or thereabouts) after surgery. I used a walker for a week after my second TKR, and a cane for the next 4 weeks. This means that any type of loose floor coverings on the stairs *that aren't securely fastened down* must go.

As you can see in the photo on the right (**Figure 8.2**), our stairwell has a very nice runner extending past the landing at the bottom. Note that the runner is securely fastened in place on each riser—a safe configuration!

In addition, throw rugs are notorious household, tripping hazards (and especially unsafe near stair landings).

<u>*The takeaway: loose floor coverings should be taken up and put away!*</u>

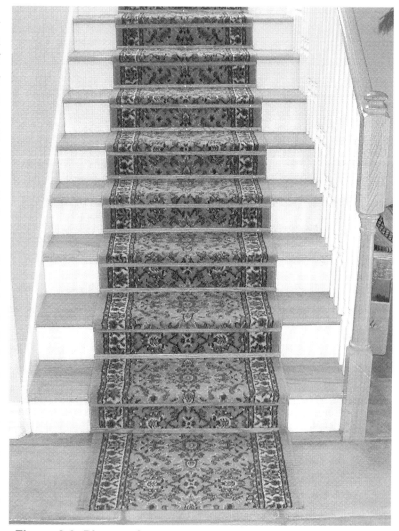

Figure 8.2 Photo of a stairwell with a securely fastened runner and sturdy handrail

94

—> <u>Watch your footing.</u> Know where your grand children and pets are at all times (especially when using the stairs) and keep all of the cute little toys picked up whenever you see them.

Little kids and pets are naturally concerned—and very loving—when they sense we're hurting—especially those wonderful, little grand children who so enrich our lives. However, both kids and/or pets can *inadvertently* cause a fall and they're both notorious for running between our feet when we least expect them to.

A good example is my black Lab—a real sweetie—she likes to go up and down the stairs with me—so I put my hand on her back and that way I always know where she's at.

<u>The takeaway: watch your footing around the house at all times!</u>

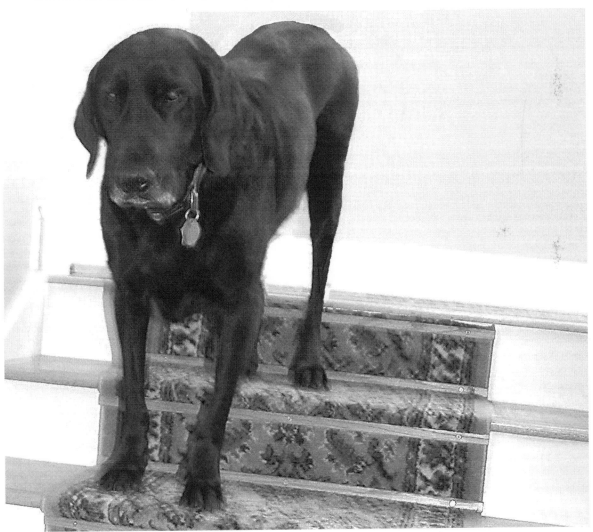

Figure 8.3 My black Lab on the stairwell is a real sweetie--but also a hazard if I don't know she's there!

—> <u>Remove tripping hazards from the floor.</u> Pick up pet dishes (and toys) to eliminate tripping hazards. Put any pet beds out of the foot traffic pattern.

Below is a photo of more floor clutter in our kitchen and it's all right at the landing for the two steps that lead to the rest of the house (**Figure 8.4**). The large dog bed, the pet dish and all of the cute, little pets toys are all potential tripping hazards. Also, I know from personal experience that stepping on a pet dish—large or small—can easily throw you off balance.

<u>The takeaway: floor clutter must be picked up and/or managed.</u>

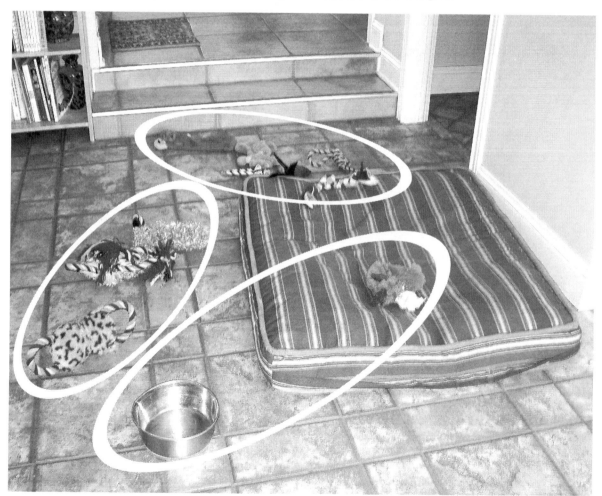

Figure 8.4 Photo showing pet toys, pet dishes and a large dog bed as examples of unsafe floor clutter

Bathrooms, Bathing and Grab Bars:

—> Install handrails and grab bars wherever they are needed.

Below is a photo of the low steps from my kitchen into the living, dining, and laundry rooms (**Figure 8.5**). I've installed a small handrail there. I also mounted an angled grab bar in the 1/2 bath adjoining our kitchen and we use it all the time.

The takeaway: consider adding grab bars and handrails in difficult to navigate areas of your home.

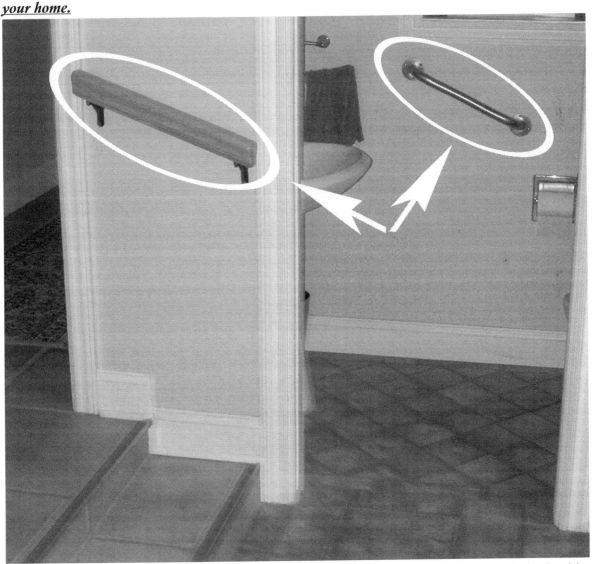

Figure 8.5 Photo of a small stairwell showing added handrail and the adjacent 1/2 bath with added grab bar

—> <u>Use an ADA-compliant bathing stool in the shower (or bathtub) to sit on safely whenever bathing.</u> Also, arrange for some help for a while after surgery.

Before my first TKR, the first thing that the occupational therapist recommended during pre-surgery orientation was to get an ADA-compliant shower-bench as depicted on the right (**Figure 8.6**). The next was to arrange to have a caregiver helping me bathe after surgery. We soon found the she was right. This little bench was indispensable and these are available almost everywhere nowadays.

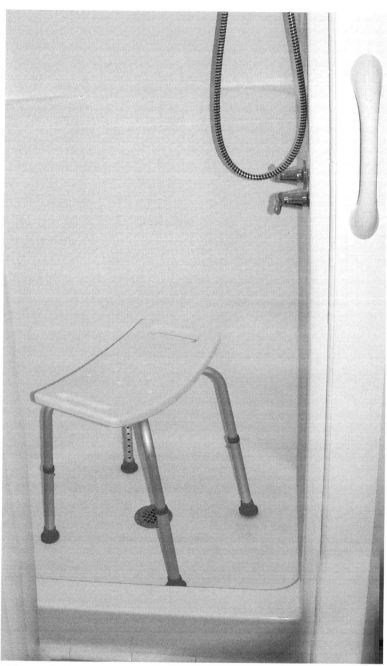

Standing in a shower can be difficult—let alone trying to bathe while following your surgeon's orders about getting the incision wet after surgery! So, if at all possible, be sure to make arrangements for somebody to help you in the shower (or tub) for at least two weeks after surgery.

Lastly—***and this is very important for hip replacement patients***—be certain to set the height to no less than nineteen inches (19"). This also works fine for knee patients like me.

<u>*The takeaway: make your shower a safe place to bathe by using a proper bathing stool and get some help for at least two weeks after surgery!*</u>

Figure 8.6 Photo of a walk-in shower with bathing stool, grab bar, and shower hose

—> <u>Create a safe environment for showering in your bathtub.</u>

Take it from me, having a nice shower after getting home from surgery is an exquisite experience, but it ought to be a safe one as well.

This is the setup we have in our hall bathroom (**Figure 8.7**). It's a good configuration for *safe showering in a bathtub* because it has a vertical grab bar (and a horizontal one too [**See Figure 8.8**]), a wire shower-caddy (for toiletries), and my grabber, which I use in case I drop something so I don't have to bend over to pick it up.

Note that all of our bathing areas have shower hose extensions. They facilitate rinsing off and mitigate the need for turning in circles when inside of a wet, slick, and soapy place. Obviously, a shower hose like this reduces the danger of slipping, or getting off-balance—bathroom falls are *dangerous*.

<u>The takeaway: setting up your bathtub to be a safe place for showering is something you'll want to do well in advance of your joint replacement surgery!</u>

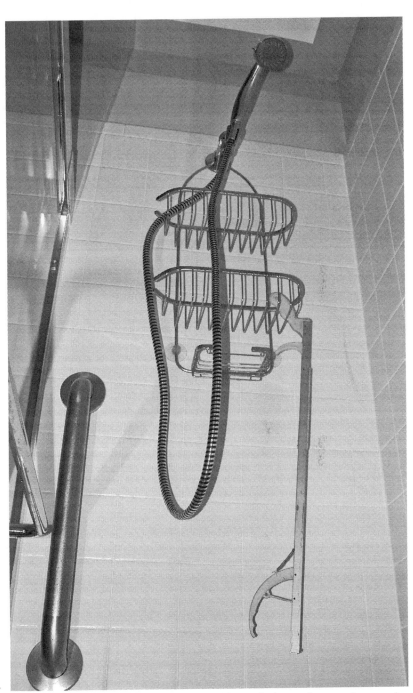

Figure 8.7 Photo of a bathtub with grab bar, shower hose attachment, shower caddy, and grabber, a safe showering setup

—> Consider placing grab bars in all of your showering and bathing areas.

Shown below (**Figure 8.8**) is an old style, cast iron tub with glass shower doors. The *handles on these shower doors are not safe grab bars*—quite the opposite! You will instinctively reach for these if you slip and you'll discover (much to your dismay) that they aren't secure at all—I found this out the hard way. It's important to note that if you already have balance problems, you should replace all towel racks and anything else in your bathroom (any and all bathing areas) that you're likely to grab for—when falling or off balance—with actual strong, safe and secure grab bars. Grab bars substitute very nicely for towel racks.

The takeaway: never assume that anything is safe to grab hold of when you're off balance! Just because things look like they're strong and secure—they may not be—and when you're already falling—it's too late.

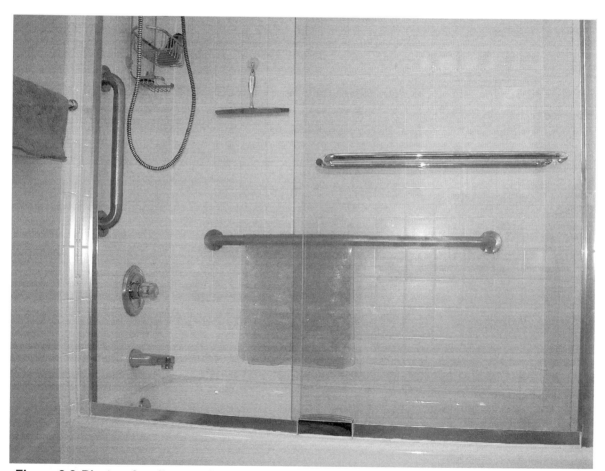

Figure 8.8 Photo of ordinary tub enclosure with shower hose, glass shower doors, vertical and horizontal grab bars, and suction-cup bathtub mat

—> <u>Grab bars and shower hoses also work for improving the bathing safety for larger tubs.</u> Secure, non-slip bath mats are also a safe addition and are recommended.

Shown below (**Figure 8.9**), is an extra-deep, extra-long tub with a shower hose and two strong grab bars. The long, horizontal grab bar is for showering safety and letting ourselves down for a bath. The vertical grab bar is for climbing in and out, which is where (and when) people are the most off balance. Note that both of these tubs are equipped with extra-large bathtub mats (with suction cups on the contact surface)—but there are many different kinds of anti-slip tub mats available.

<u>The takeaway: whether it's a large tub, a regular tub, or a walk-in shower—all can be made safe for joint replacement patients—and the rest of the family too!</u>

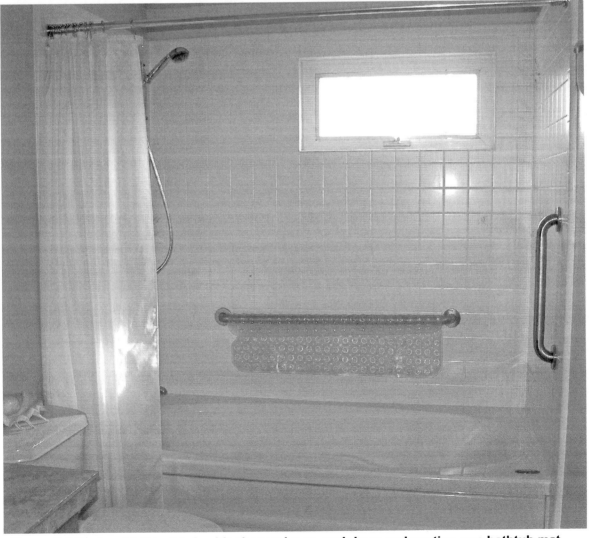

Figure 8.9 Photo of tall bathtub with shower hose, grab bars and suction-cup bathtub mat

—> Take steps to make sure your toilets are adequate and safe for your type of surgery!

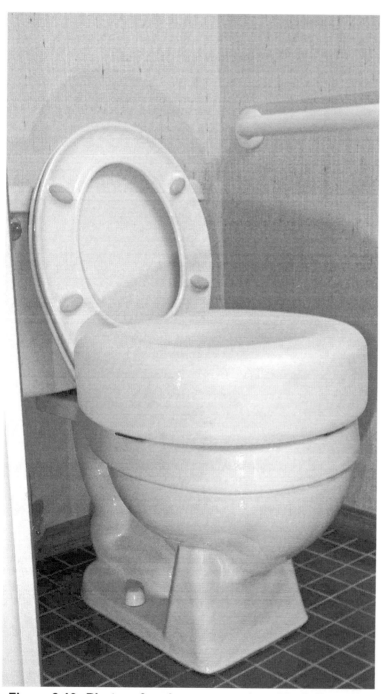

Here is an example of a standard, 14" high commode (**Figure 8.10**). Note that a generic toilet seat extender has been installed to raise up the seat height to 19". This makes this old commode safe for a hip replacement patient because it's been transformed to the minimum height.

You can purchase an inexpensive, generic, toilet seat extender almost anywhere these days. More elaborate ones can be found at a durable, medical supply store (or can be ordered from the Internet), some of them come with hand rails, some can actually be fastened to the commode, and some even have arms and legs like an easy chair.

Your occupational therapist can help you determine what's best for you.

The takeaway: your toilet must be high enough (at least 19") to be safe for your hip replacement!

Figure 8.10 Photo of a low commode with toilet seat extender added for hip or even knee replacement patients

Hugate's Comment: *Your toilet seats must not be less than 19" high (as measured from the floor to the top of the seat). For most hip replacement patients, the average toilet seat is too low and I recommend a toilet seat extender (**Figure 8.10**). One of these will augment your current toilet seat so that it's high enough to be safe.*

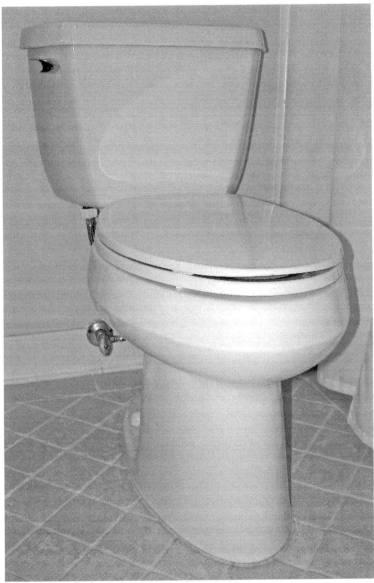

Figure 8.11 Photo of an ADA-compliant commode

Alternatively, you could have an ADA-compliant toilet installed like the one depicted here (**Figure 8.11**). However, it is my recommendation that if you are a hip replacement patient, please make sure your new commode is at least 19" high. ~*~

On the left (**Figure 8.11**), we show an example of a very nice, ADA-compliant commode. We have these throughout our home. This leads to the question:

What is the difference between an ADA-compliant unit versus a standard commode?

Basically, most toilets come in two, fundamental shapes (round and elongated), but ADA commodes are required to be elongated and taller (17"-19" high) than their standard counterparts.

103

This brings us to a close on preparing your home for joint replacement recovery. Our objective here is not to create a complete list of everything you can do to prepare your home after your joint replacement surgery, but rather to show some common sense examples and to get you to thinking of ways you can make those first few weeks (and the rest of your life for that matter) easier and safer. Remember, you have local, neighborhood resources who can assist you in evaluating your home and possibly even finding financial resources depending on your situation. So don't be afraid to go to your library, city offices, county outreach program, state outreach program, local senior center, or your religious institution and ask them to help you locate resources in your community.

I wish you a safe and uneventful recovery.

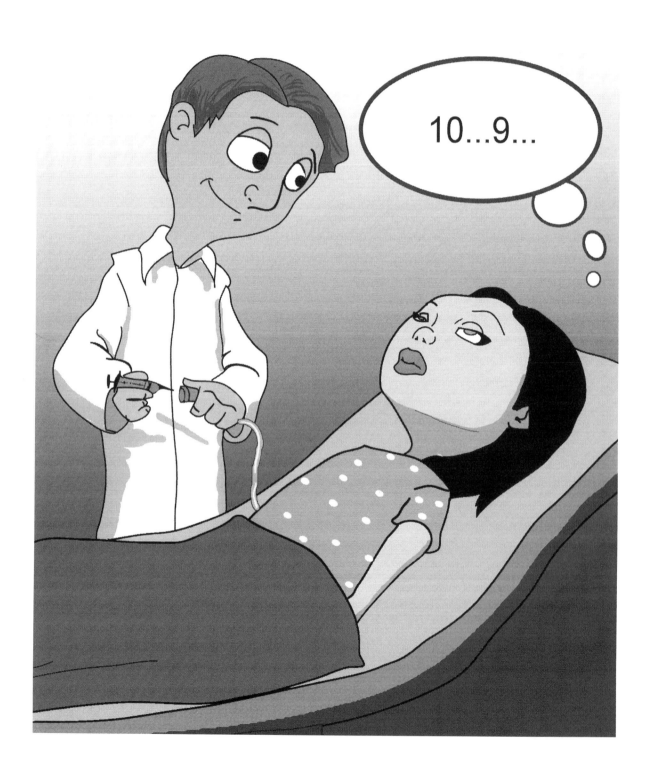

Anesthesia Options in Joint Replacement Surgery

CHAPTER 9

by Dr. Giancarlo Checa

For many patients, anesthesia is one of the most significant concerns when considering surgery. For some it is the fear of "losing control" of what's going on which fuels the worry. For others the major concern is medical: "Will I ever wake up?" These anxieties are understandable and are *normal*! You'll be delighted to know, however, that undergoing anesthesia is very safe for the vast majority of patients these days. The risks vary, of course, depending on what medical problems you may have before surgery. Your initial conversations regarding your anesthesia risk will be with your surgeon. A careful assessment of your health status will be a major part of the conversation with your surgeon as you discuss the decision to have joint replacement surgery.

Hugate's Comment: For this chapter of our handbook, I've invited my good friend and talented colleague Dr. Gianni Checa to describe the anesthesia experience to you. As we explained in the introduction, this book is all about educating you, the reader, through different perspectives. Dr. Checa is a board certified anesthesiologist with additional fellowship training in pain management techniques. His perspective will prove to be valuable to you. Dr. Checa will add a layer of detail to the subject and in the process answer many of the questions about anesthesia that may be floating around in your head. Interestingly, many of my patients are more anxious about having anesthesia than they are about having the surgery itself. Dr. Checa does a great job of describing your options and putting into perspective the risks associated with anesthesia.

As with all of our contributors, Dr. Checa describes his methods and opinions here. While there are many anesthesia options that lead to a good result, the decision about your anesthetic should be based on a number of personal factors and would be an individual decision made by you and your anesthesiologist. Use this information as a guide to what options are available and what questions to ask during the preoperative discussion with your anesthesiologist. ~*~

Generally, if you're relatively healthy, with no chronic medical conditions, or if you have medical conditions that are well controlled, you're a good candidate for anesthesia. In fact, driving your car for a year is over forty times more likely to result in a fatality than undergoing anesthesia. A 1999 report by the Institute of Medicine indicated that anesthesia care is nearly fifty times safer now than it was in the 1980s (when anesthesia was already considered very safe). One of the first things I try to do when meeting with patients is to put things in perspective for them, and generally speaking, when people hear these statistics, they feel a sense of relief.

To make sure that anesthesia will be as safe as possible for you, your surgeon and/ or PCP may order preoperative testing. The most common preoperative assessments are blood work to check your overall health status, a chest X-ray to assess your lungs, and an EKG to verify your heart health. Patients with chronic heart or lung problems may be asked to complete a more in-depth medical workup that includes a heart stress test or lung function tests. On occasion, patients with complex preoperative medical problems may need to see a cardiologist (heart specialist) or a pulmonologist (lung specialist) to assess their risk for surgery. Your surgeon, PCP, and anesthesiologist will review these tests to make sure that you're a good candidate to receive anesthesia. In addition to determining if you're a candidate for surgery, these test results can also be used to determine the *safest* type of anesthesia for you.

During your joint surgery you'll be cared for by an anesthesia provider. Your anesthesia provider will either be an anesthesiologist, or a nurse anesthetist. Anesthesiologists are physicians (either medical doctors or doctors of osteopathy) who have completed medical school and a four year residency program with a specialty in anesthesia. All anesthesiologists are licensed through their state board of medicine, and most maintain specialty certification through the American Board of Anesthesiology. A certified, registered nurse anesthetist (CRNA) is an advanced practice registered nurse who has graduate level training and board certification in the specialty of anesthesia. CRNAs are licensed through their state board of nursing and the Council for Certification of Nurse Anesthetists. Both anesthesiologists and CRNAs can provide excellent anesthesia care.

In most cases, if your provider is a CRNA, he'll be under the direct supervision of an anesthesiologist.

Your anesthesia provider takes care of you throughout the perioperative period. The perioperative period consists of the time spent in the preoperative holding area, during surgery, and in the surgical recovery room. The role of the anesthesia provider is two-fold: to control your pain and discomfort, and also make sure your body adjusts well to the anesthetic during surgery. Most patients will meet their anesthesiologist for the first time on the day of surgery. However, some patients, and especially those with a significant chronic medical condition or a previous adverse reaction to anesthesia, may speak to (or meet) their anesthesiologist prior to surgery. If you've had any bad experiences with anesthesia in the past, are especially concerned about anesthesia, or feel that you have medical conditions that may make anesthesia more difficult for you, talk to your surgeon. Your surgeon will help you decide if you need to speak with your anesthesiologist in advance of surgery.

The Night Before Surgery

To make your joint replacement surgery as safe as possible, most patients are asked not to eat or drink anything after midnight the evening before their surgery. It's important that your stomach is empty when surgery begins because this decreases the risk of aspirating (breathing in your stomach contents while under anesthesia). While aspiration is an uncommon event, it's important to take every precaution to avoid it. Sometimes, if your surgery is scheduled later in the day, you may have food up to eight hours before your surgery begins and water or other clear liquids up to six hours beforehand—but check with your surgeon or anesthesiologist first. Clear liquids include Sprite, 7-Up, cranberry juice, apple juice, or coffee or tea *without cream or milk.* In general any liquid you can hold in a glass and see through is considered a "clear liquid." If you don't follow these guidelines, your surgery may be delayed or rescheduled for your safety.

If you're on medication, your surgeon will let you know which medications to take on the morning of your surgery. If you have contact with your anesthesiologist prior to the day of surgery, he will also help you determine which medications to take. When you take your medications on the morning of surgery, please use the smallest possible sip of water needed to get the pills down. The following is a very general set of medication guidelines. Remember, your surgeon, anesthesiologist, or PCP must make the final decision about what preoperative medications are right for you.

On the Day of Surgery

In general, you SHOULD NOT take:

- *Any medication that states "take with food or milk" on the label.*
- *Large bulk medications such as Metamucil (dietary fiber).*
- *Diabetes medication that you take by mouth.*
- *Diuretics (water pills) except in rare cases.*
- *Blood thinners (such as Coumadin, Aspirin, Plavix, Lovenox), and other Nonsteroidal Anti-Inflammatory agents (such as Motrin, Advil, ibuprofen, Naprosyn) should be stopped as directed by your surgeon.*
- *Call your surgeon's office if you usually take any of these medicines and have received no specific instructions.*
- *Take only those herbal or natural medications approved by your surgeon or anesthesiologist.*

In general, you SHOULD take:

- *Chronic pain medications (other than those listed above)*
- *Insulin: Your dose for the day of surgery may be determined by your surgeon, anesthesiologist, or PCP.*
- *Inhalers for asthma and emphysema: use as scheduled and bring your inhalers with you to the hospital for continued use during hospitalization.*

It's best to wear glasses rather than contacts to the hospital and to leave all of your jewelry at home. If you're more comfortable wearing some of your jewelry (your wedding ring, for example) to the hospital, please make sure that you have someone you can leave it with right before surgery. You will not be able to wear any jewelry during surgery and the hospital will not be responsible for lost or stolen valuables. It's best to wear your hair loose (without hairpins or rubber bands) because you'll have to remove these items prior to surgery. Some patients choose to wear makeup to surgery. This is not a problem; however, it usually becomes smudged during the surgical process. If you wear fingernail polish to surgery, be aware that the anesthesiologist may have to remove fingernail polish from one nail to properly monitor your oxygen levels.

If you're one of the few patients who forgoes general anesthesia and remains awake for surgery (with a nerve block and mild sedation), you may want to bring an iPod or other device so you can listen to music or guided meditation during surgery.

Different Stops on the Day of Surgery

The Preoperative Area

After admission to the hospital or surgery center, you'll be taken to the preoperative holding area. You may have a supportive friend or family member accompany you to the preoperative area and remain with you until you're taken into the operating room. You'll meet your anesthesiologist here in the preoperative area. Your anesthesiologist, along with your preoperative nurse, will talk to you about your current health, your health history, and your previous experience with anesthesia. It is especially important to bring a list of all of your medications (including natural and herbal supplements) and to mention any allergies that you may have. Your anesthesiologist will also do a basic physical exam and evaluate your vital signs. Here your preoperative testing is reviewed as well.

Please let your anesthesiologist know if you have a pacemaker. Don't worry: most patients with pacemakers will not need any type of extra interventions. If you have a defibrillator (AICD), be sure to ask your cardiologist if you need to have it reprogrammed before and after surgery. Some defibrillators do need to be reprogrammed and others don't. Your surgeon and anesthesiologist should be made aware that you have a defibrillator as well.

After carefully considering the nature of your surgery, your current and past health history, the results of your preoperative tests, and your own concerns and preferences, you (the patient), your anesthesiologist, and your surgeon will make the final decision about the type of anesthesia that's best and safest for you. Your anesthesiologist will review the risks and benefits of your anesthesia plan with you and obtain your informed consent for anesthesia care. He'll be able to answer questions about your anesthesia as well as questions about the monitoring and management of your medical conditions during surgery. If you have questions or concerns about anesthesia, be sure to write them down before coming to the hospital—this makes them easier to remember. It's important to have all of your questions answered and be comfortable with your anesthesia plan prior to beginning surgery.

Hugate's Comment: This is also a great time to let your anesthesia provider know if you have issues with nausea. Most people who are having joint replacement surgery have had surgery in the past. If your prior experiences with anesthesia or pain medications included severe nausea, let the anesthesiologist know. They have a number of preemptive tools to prevent this from becoming a problem. Depending on the severity, a tendency toward nausea may even influence which type of anesthesia you undergo. I encourage you to put this on your written list of questions for your anesthesiologist so you don't forget to bring it up. Severe nausea will not only make you miserable after surgery, it can also slow down your recovery and rehabilitation. ~*~

While in the preoperative area, you'll be prepared for surgery. You'll be asked to completely undress, and your clothes and other belongings will be securely stored for you. You'll also be asked to remove your jewelry (including your wedding ring), your eyeglasses or contacts, and your dentures. You may wait to remove your dentures until right before leaving the preoperative area. You'll also need to remove your hearing aids. Your hearing aids will be removed either immediately before going to the operating room or by your anesthesiologist once you're asleep.

Hugate's Comment: Why do we have you remove all jewelry? There are a couple of reasons. First, during the surgery we use an electro-cautery device to dissect through tissues with minimal blood loss. It uses electricity to "burn" the small blood vessels and prevent bleeding. If you have a piece of metallic jewelry and that jewelry hits a piece of grounded metal, you could sustain a burn from the electro-cautery "shorting" out.

The other issue here is that of swelling. Suppose you have a tight wedding band on your finger and undergo surgery. During the surgery, you get fluids through your veins (known as intravenous or IV fluids) and this may cause your fingers to swell. If your finger swells too much, you may not be able to remove the ring for a few days. Further, if the ring strangulates the swollen finger, you could damage the finger. You could also lose your jewelry during all the "action" while you're in the hospital. For these reasons we generally discourage the wearing of jewelry during surgery. it's just easier to leave it at home. ~*~

Your preoperative nurse will start an IV, most likely in your arm, and begin infusing fluids. This is the IV that your anesthesiologist will use to administer your anesthetic and other medications during your surgery. Some patients may need an additional IV line once in the operating room. If you have significant heart problems, you may receive an arterial blood pressure catheter (similar to an IV but placed in an artery instead of a vein) in your wrist area. This special type of catheter may be put into place in the preoperative area or in the operating room. It allows the anesthesiologist to monitor your blood pressure constantly instead of intermittently (every few minutes) as it would typically be with a blood pressure cuff.

There are two broad categories of anesthesia that one can use to undergo joint replacements, *general anesthesia* and *regional anesthesia*. Most people who undergo hip or knee replacement surgery will have general anesthesia. General anesthesia is the use of intravenous medications and/or anesthetic gasses to put you to "sleep" for the surgery. You will not remember anything that happens while you're under general anesthesia and you will not be aware of the sensation of pain. This is what most people think of when they think of *anesthesia*.

Some patients receive regional anesthesia during their joint replacement surgery, either by itself with mild sedation, or *in addition to* general anesthesia. Regional anesthesia (frequently called a "nerve block") is the injection of medications near specific nerves to make those nerves numb and to decrease or eliminate the sensation of pain in certain areas of your body. Although regional anesthesia can be used to provide pain relief during the surgery itself, the major advantage of regional anesthesia is the ability to control pain in the hours and days after surgery. As such, many patients undergoing joint replacement surgery may receive some sort of regional anesthesia. In general, there are more regional anesthetic options for knee replacement patients than hip replacement patients.

While specific types of regional anesthesia will be discussed in greater detail later in this chapter, it's important to mention it here because most regional anesthesia is administered before surgery begins.

113

The anesthesiologist will sometimes perform a nerve block in the preoperative area before a patient enters the operating room, or in a special room designated for placing nerve blocks called a "block room." The anesthesiologist may also administer medication in your IV in the preoperative area to make you less anxious during the placement of the nerve block. While this medication will not put you to sleep like general anesthesia, it will help you to relax and may even cause you to forget some things that happen after it's administered.

The Operating Room

When it's time for your surgery to begin, you'll be wheeled into the operating room. Once in the operating room, you'll be transferred onto the operating table. If you're going to receive a nerve block prior to surgery, and it wasn't administered in the preoperative area, it'll be placed now. You'll then lie down on the operating table and the anesthesiologist or operative nurse will apply several different monitors to your body to assess your vital signs throughout the procedure. A blood pressure cuff will be placed on one of your arms, an oxygen saturation monitor will be placed on one of your fingers, and EKG pads will be placed on your chest and the sides of your rib cage. None of these monitors will cause you any discomfort or pain, and they will provide your anesthesiologist with essential information during your surgery. An *oxygen mask* will be placed over your nose and mouth. The extra oxygen you receive through this mask helps prepare your body for anesthesia and you'll continue to breathe normally while your oxygen mask is on.

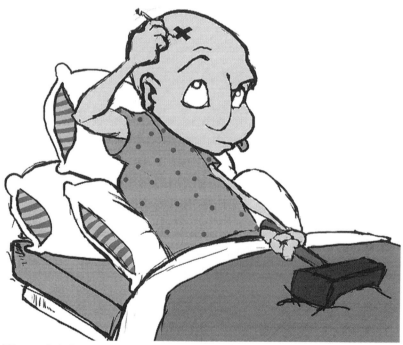

Figure 9.1 Cartoon "Never mind the anesthesia, Doc! I'll take of it!"

114

After all of your monitors and oxygen mask are in place, your anesthesiologist will administer medication through your IV to help you relax (if he has not already done so). If you opted for general anesthesia, the anesthesiologist will now administer medication that will cause you to go to sleep. These medications work very quickly. Many people like to focus on relaxing and positive thoughts as they go to sleep. After you're fully asleep, the anesthesiologist will insert a breathing tube into your windpipe. You will not feel the breathing tube go in or even remember it. The breathing tube will stay in through the remainder of your surgery. Your anesthesiologist will continuously monitor your well-being throughout your surgery and make sure that you're sleeping and that your pain is well controlled.

<u>*The Post Anesthesia Care Unit (Recovery Room)*</u>

Once your surgery is complete, your anesthesiologist will wake you and take you to the surgical recovery room, sometimes called the PACU (post-anesthesia care unit). Because of the medications in your system, you will not remember waking up in the operating room or even the trip to the recovery room. Some patients won't remember their stay in the recovery room either. When you arrive in the recovery room you will get a new blood pressure cuff, oxygen saturation monitor, and heart monitors. Your vital signs will be monitored closely by the recovery room nurses. The recovery room nurses will also help you manage any postoperative pain, nausea, or itching that you may have. An anesthesiologist will always be available to assist the nurses with your care if needed.

Most patients stay in the recovery room for about an hour to an hour and a half after joint replacement surgery. Once your breathing, blood oxygen level, level of consciousness (how awake you are), blood pressure, and ability to move meet certain criteria, you'll be moved to your hospital room on the orthopedic care unit of your hospital or surgery center.

Options in Anesthesia

That was a general description of what the typical anesthesia experience may be for you. As I have mentioned several times, there are a number of options available. However, not every option is a good choice for every patient. Let's take some time now and go over the standard options available to most joint replacement patients today. Again, the most appropriate anesthetic for you is an individual decision that takes into account a number of issues. If there are no major medical issues that dictate your anesthetic, it usually boils down to preference, your preference, and that of the surgeon and anesthesiologist. In the following pages we'll examine these options in much greater detail, dispel any misconception you might have and illuminate your choices.

Hugate's Comment: *Another factor in what anesthetic options you may have is the skill set of your anesthesia provider. Dr. Checa is well versed in a number of regional anesthetic techniques because of his training. I choose to work with anesthesiologists who have a "big bag of tricks," meaning they're able to offer a number of different anesthetic options. Every anesthesiologist has her comfort zone, however, and I don't recommend that you ask for an anesthetic that your provider isn't completely comfortable administering. ~*~*

Overview: General Anesthesia

General anesthesia is the most common anesthetic choice for both hip and knee replacement surgery. When under general anesthesia, patients are completely "asleep." They're not aware of what is happening and they don't experience any pain. Patients who elect general anesthesia for their surgery have no memory of the surgery and may not remember the events immediately preceding or following the administration of the general anesthetic.

General anesthesia is usually administered both through IV medications and through anesthetic gases that you breathe. Once you're fully asleep, a breathing tube will be placed. This tube will extend from your mouth to either your throat or your trachea (windpipe). Because the breathing tube may cause you to gag when placed, it's very important to have an empty stomach prior to surgery (as we discussed earlier). Having an empty stomach will decrease the risk of your stomach contents being aspirated (or inhaled) into the lungs. Once the breathing tube is placed, it'll be hooked up to a ventilator (breathing machine) which will deliver oxygen and anesthetic gasses. Your breathing tube will be removed once you begin to awaken afterward. You may have a slightly sore throat for several days after having a breathing tube. Drinking warm liquids and using throat lozenges are usually the best way to manage this type of postoperative discomfort.

Other than a sore throat, the most common side effect from general anesthesia is postoperative nausea and vomiting (PONV). Fortunately, the medications and techniques used in anesthesia today have dramatically reduced the incidence of PONV. You will most likely be given medication during your surgery to combat PONV, and anti-nausea medication will also be available for you in the recovery room and in your hospital room too. Much less common adverse reactions to general anesthesia include an allergic reaction to the anesthetic medication and heart problems. However, heart problems are extremely uncommon and are only a significant concern in patients who aren't healthy. Again, your health status at the time of surgery plays the biggest role in determining your anesthetic risk. And remember our discussion at the beginning of the chapter: if you're relatively healthy, you're over forty times more likely to die by driving a car for a year than from receiving general anesthesia.

Overview: Regional Anesthesia

Many patients who have hip or knee replacement surgery will receive *regional anesthesia*, sometimes called a "nerve block." Regional anesthesia is most frequently used to provide pain control *after* the surgery is over. However, some patients choose to have their surgery using a nerve block alone and **without going to sleep** under general anesthesia. These patients will receive regional anesthesia with intravenous sedation in lieu of general anesthesia.

Regional anesthesia is a method of blocking pain signals from reaching your brain. When the body experiences an injury (or surgery), a pain signal is generated in the nerve closest to the site of the surgery. The pain signal then travels through the nerve, up the spinal cord, and to the brain. When the brain receives the signal from the nerve, it interprets the signal as pain. It's only after the brain decodes the nerve transmission that you become aware of your pain. When you're under

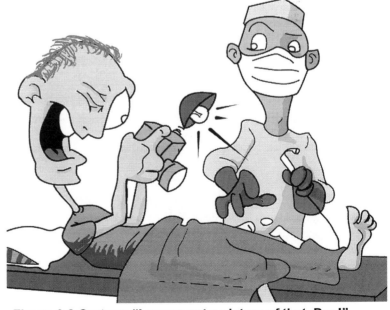

Figure 9.2 Cartoon "Lemme get a picture of that, Doc!"

general anesthesia, your brain is asleep and unable to interpret the pain signals being sent by your body. Regional anesthesia stops the signals *before* they reach the brain by blocking the signals in the nerves.

Regional anesthesia can be divided into two main categories: central and peripheral. *Central regional anesthesia* provides a way of blocking the pain signal at the level of the spine. The pain signal is generated at the site of the surgery and is transmitted through local nerves (the nerves of your hip or knee) to the spinal cord. The central regional anesthetic block numbs the nerves in the spinal cord so that the pain signal stops there and never reaches the brain. Because the pain message is blocked before the brain can receive it, the brain doesn't register the pain message and you don't feel any pain.

Peripheral regional anesthesia works in a similar fashion. The difference is that peripheral regional anesthesia blocks the transmission of the pain before it even gets to the spinal cord, usually very close to the site where the pain is generated. For example, if you have knee replacement surgery, the pain signal is blocked at the nerves immediately surrounding the knee and never travels to the spinal cord. This process is similar to "local anesthesia" which is used to numb small areas of the body like your mouth prior to dental work. However, peripheral regional anesthesia blocks nerves that control much larger areas of the body. The end result of peripheral regional anesthesia is the same as that of central regional anesthesia: the pain signal never reaches the brain and you don't experience any pain. We'll discuss specific regional blocks a little later on.

Regional Anesthesia with Sedation

There are a few different reasons why some patients don't receive general anesthesia at all for their hip or knee replacement surgery. Some patients have had a previous difficult experience with being put to sleep. Others have medical conditions that may increase the risk of general anesthesia. Sometimes patients have a significant fear of general anesthesia or of "losing control" when being put to sleep. Any of these reasons may make you a good candidate to have surgery with a combination of regional anesthesia and IV sedation. The decision to avoid general anesthesia is one you make in conjunction with your surgeon and anesthesiologist. If you have concerns about undergoing general anesthesia, and you feel like an alternate option may be right for you, discuss these concerns with your surgeon early in the decision making process.

If you're considering surgery without general anesthesia, your primary question is most likely "will I feel any pain?" The answer is no. Regional anesthesia will prevent you from feeling pain during your surgery. Still, while you will not experience pain during your surgical procedure, you probably don't think of surgery as an opportunity to relax and unwind! Almost everyone approaches surgery with some apprehension, and, for most people, being aware of the surgical process as it occurs doesn't help alleviate the anxiety. This is why intravenous sedation is administered in conjunction with regional anesthesia in patients who don't receive general anesthesia.

Intravenous sedation (also called "conscious sedation" and "twilight anesthesia") allows you to become very relaxed and sleepy, and you may even fall asleep. Unlike general anesthesia, however, twilight anesthesia is similar to a very relaxed natural sleep state—you will not be unconscious and you're able to respond to verbal requests (perhaps with some light prodding). While some people will remember what happens while they're under IV sedation, most will not have any memory of the experience at all. The primary risk associated with IV sedation is a possible (but very rare) allergic reaction to the medication that's used. The advantage of IV sedation is that you wake up relatively quickly and easily. Also, most people don't feel nauseated or have significant lingering effects of any kind.

Regional Anesthesia and Postoperative Pain Control

There are two commonly used postoperative pain control methods: pain medications and regional anesthesia. Pain medications are usually given through an IV in the first hours or days following surgery. Once your pain has decreased, your surgeon will prescribe pain pills to take by mouth instead of the IV pain medications. The pain medication that's given through your IV may cause several side effects. The most common side effects include drowsiness, dizziness, lightheadedness, nausea, vomiting, itching, constipation, and difficulty urinating. Rarely, your IV pain medication may cause you to get extremely sleepy and slow your breathing rate. Your level of alertness and breathing will be monitored very closely if you're given IV pain medication. While IV pain medication can dramatically decrease postoperative pain in the first hours and days following surgery, it usually doesn't provide total pain relief, especially immediately following your operative procedure.

The second option for postoperative pain relief is regional anesthesia. If used for postoperative pain relief, regional anesthesia can be given in conjunction with general anesthesia. Regional anesthesia enables you to experience excellent postoperative pain relief (usually more complete relief than that experienced with IV pain medications alone) without the potential side effects of IV pain medications. However, there are some side effects that can occur with regional anesthesia as well.

119

Holland's Comment: When I had my first TKR, I didn't have the regional anesthesia or "nerve block." Even before this first TKR, we knew I was allergic to certain pain medications. As a result, after surgery we had a very difficult time finding pain medications that worked for me without causing significant, unwanted side effects. One of these caused me to break out in itchy red bumps that lasted for about two weeks, which also necessitated that I take a powerful, oral antihistamine.

This can be exhausting for you as the patient. It was beyond exhausting for me. It takes the body time to discover which pain medication will work. If a pain medication isn't alleviating your pain, it takes some time clear from your system (or wear off) before another medication can be tried. Then, of course, you're still in pain while this next medication takes its own sweet time to begin alleviating your pain, and then it may not be effective either—"Sheesh!" In the meantime (emphasis on "mean") there you lay—and there I lay—suffering through several trial-and-error loops for almost two days before the pain began to settle down to tolerable levels. This was not fun!

When Dr. Hugate performed my second TKR, we had my first experience to draw from and I chose to have a regional block—the femoral nerve block with a catheter—as well as the general anesthetic. I urge you to consider such a nerve block as Dr. Checa describes here. The difference between these two TKR experiences was different as night and day—the second TKR was a breeze by comparison to the first. Regional anesthesia can make all the difference during your post-operative hospital stay. ~*~

Specific Regional Anesthesia Techniques

Spinal Anesthesia

Spinal anesthesia, commonly called a "spinal," is a form of nerve block where the spinal nerves are blocked at their roots. Because it blocks the nerves at the level of the spine, it's a *central regional anesthetic.* Spinals are usually administered in the operating room before surgery begins. Many patients are given light intravenous sedation before the spinal is placed to minimize any anxiety they may have. The sedation may also cause you to forget the spinal placement procedure ever happened. The nurse or anesthesiologist will help you get into a position that allows the anesthesiologist to place the spinal in the correct location (you'll be seated with your back rounded out and your shoulders slumped over, or lying on your side). Once you're positioned, the anesthesiologist will clean off your back with an antiseptic (this may feel cold) and place a drape to keep the area clean. He will then use a very small needle to inject numbing medication into the skin of your back where he will place the spinal. This numbing medication stings, but the discomfort lasts for less than a minute. Once the numbing medication takes effect, you will not feel any more pain for the rest of the spinal placement procedure.

A longer needle will then be placed into your back and through the tissues between your backbones. When this needle is placed, you may feel pressure in your back, but you shouldn't feel any pain. Your backbones surround and protect your spinal cord (which is the column of nerves that sends signals back and forth between your body and your brain). The spinal cord is housed in a sack composed of protective, connective tissue coverings, the outermost of which is called the dura. This sack courses down the center of your back bones and is filled with fluid that bathes the spinal cord and the brain with nutrients. The needle is placed through the sack, but *not* into the spinal cord. Medication (usually a numbing medication and a narcotic pain medication) will be injected into this fluid. The medication numbs the nerves coming from the lower part of your spinal cord. This numbing prevents pain signals from the lower half of your body (your toes to your belly) from being transmitted up the spinal cord and, hence, to the brain. Because the brain doesn't receive the pain signals, you will not experience any pain.

After your spinal is placed, your legs will start to feel very heavy and numb. Within a few minutes you lose the ability to feel anything that's touching the lower half of your body, and you will not be able to move anything below your belly button. If your spinal is being used for pain control during surgery in lieu of general anesthesia, the surgeon will make sure that you're completely numb before beginning the operation. If your spinal is placed for surgical pain control only, the numbness begins to wear off about four hours after it's placed and definitely *after* your surgery is complete. If your spinal has been placed for postoperative pain control, it will likely include a long-acting pain medication. This medication will give you pain relief for up to twenty-four hours following placement of the spinal.

The most common side effects of spinal anesthesia are low blood pressure (which the anesthesiologist can correct by giving you medication through your IV) and soreness where the needle was placed. Uncommon risks include headache (less than 3 percent of patients will get a headache), bleeding into the injection site, infection of the injection site, and nerve injury. Permanent nerve function problems are very rare and occur in about 1 out of every 220,000 patients who have spinal anesthesia. If you receive long-acting pain medication in your spinal you may experience itching after you wake up from surgery.

121

If you do begin to itch, let your nurse know right away and he can give you medication that will correct the problem.

Epidural Anesthesia

Epidural anesthesia is the second form of central regional anesthesia. An epidural injection works very similarly to a spinal: it numbs the nerves that send pain signals back and forth between the lower half of the body and the brain. However, if you receive an epidural injection, the medication is placed in a slightly different location than it would be during spinal anesthesia. As you recall, when a spinal is placed, the medication is injected through the dura and into the fluid that surrounds the spinal cord. When an epidural is placed, the needle stops just short of the dura—it doesn't go through it. The medications (usually a numbing medicine and a narcotic pain medicine) are then injected into the epidural space located between the dura and the backbone. The epidural medication is able to numb the same nerves that the spinal anesthetic affects. Pain relief is likewise accomplished through blocking the transmission of pain signals in these nerves as the pain makes its way to the brain.

From the patient's perspective, the epidural placement procedure feels very much like the procedure used to place a spinal. While the spinal is always administered as a single dose of medication, the epidural can be given as either a single dose or through the use of an *epidural catheter*. An epidural catheter is a very small flexible plastic tube that's inserted through the needle which is placed into the epidural space. This tube is then left in the epidural space after the needle is removed. The epidural catheter is similar to the small tube that's left in your vein when an IV is placed. You won't feel the catheter in your back and it shouldn't cause you any discomfort. The catheter allows medication to be continuously pumped into the epidural space so pain control can be maintained for as long as necessary.

If you received a single dose of medication into the epidural space, your pain control, numbness, and inability to move will wear off about four hours after your epidural was placed. However, if a long-acting pain medication is injected into the epidural space, you can have up to twenty-four hours of pain relief. Patients who have a catheter placed in the epidural space experience excellent pain control for as long as the catheter is in place and connected to a medication pump. Following hip and knee replacement surgery, most patients who have an epidural catheter receive pain medication through their catheter for approximately two to three days following surgery. The catheter removal will not be painful—most patients don't feel it at all.

The side effects associated with epidural anesthesia are very similar to those experienced with spinal anesthesia. The most common side effects of epidural anesthesia are low blood pressure (which the anesthesiologist can correct by giving you medication through your IV), unequal pain control (one side of your body is more numb than the other), and soreness where the needle was placed. Relatively rare risks include headache (about 1 percent of patients will get a headache), bleeding into the injection site (affecting approximately 1 in 168,000 patients), infection of the injection site (affecting approximately 1 in 145,000 patients), and non-permanent nerve injury (affecting approximately 1 in 6,700 patients). Permanent nerve function problems are very rare and occur in 1 out of every 150,000 patients who have epidural anesthesia. If you receive a long-acting epidural pain medication, you may experience itching after you awaken from surgery. If you do begin to itch, let your nurse know right away and he can give you medication that will correct the problem.

Peripheral Nerve Block

There are three main peripheral nerve blocks used for hip and/or knee replacement surgery: *lumbar plexus blocks*, *femoral nerve blocks*, and *sciatic nerve blocks*. Like spinal and epidural anesthesia, peripheral nerve blocks can provide pain relief both during and after surgery. When a peripheral nerve block is placed, medication is injected near a nerve that's outside of the spinal column and closer to the area of the body that needs to be numbed. The advantage of peripheral nerve blocks over central nerve blocks is that the anesthesiologist is able to numb a smaller and more specific region of the body. However, peripheral nerve blocks require a greater level of expertise, and not all anesthesiologists can perform them. There are several uncommon side effects associated with peripheral nerve blocks, including infection, a buildup of blood near the nerve (hematoma), nerve injury, and accidental injection of medication into the blood vessels.

The peripheral nerve block placement procedure is very similar to the spinal and epidural procedures that we've discussed; however, these blocks include an extra step. Everyone's body is unique, and once the nerves leave the spinal column, they travel along slightly different paths in each individual patient. Therefore, the anesthesiologist will either use an *ultrasound picture* or a *nerve stimulator* to find out exactly where your nerves are located. An ultrasound machine allows the anesthesiologist to see different structures inside your body including your nerves. The ultrasound doesn't use any radiation to create the picture (only sound waves), it has no known side effects, and is painless. The ultrasound wand will be covered with a clear jelly (which may feel cold), and the anesthesiologist will glide the wand over your skin to locate the nerve underneath. Once they locate the nerve, the injection needle is placed next to the nerve, and the numbing medication injected.

If your anesthesiologist instead uses a nerve stimulator to find your nerve, he will place a small needle through your skin in the area where the nerve is expected to be. This needle is attached to a nerve stimulator machine that generates a very small electrical current. The electrical current will stimulate the nerve and cause your muscle to twitch, and the closer the current comes to the nerve, the more it will twitch. This lets the anesthesiologist know that the needle is in the correct location. Once your anesthesiologist has found the correct spot (close to the nerve), he will inject numbing medication into the space through the same needle that delivers the electrical current. The idea of an electrical current being passed through a needle and into your nerve sounds rather frightening; however, you will not experience any pain with this procedure. The amount of electricity used is extremely small. Some people find the nerve stimulator slightly uncomfortable, but most perceive it as a "strange" or "funny" feeling. The nerve stimulator machine itself is not associated with any known side effects or safety risks.

Holland's Comment: While working on this chapter, Dr. Hugate asked me if I remember receiving the procedure Dr. Checa details above, with the nerve stimulator to guide the placement of the specialized nerve block catheter.

In truth, my recollections are vague, but I do remember. By this time in the process, my anesthesiologist had already given me the medication to help me be calm, but I remember the feeling of him searching for the nerve to place the catheter—which is an exceedingly narrow catheter much smaller than an IV. I especially recall the strange feeling Dr. Checa describes. It was not painful, but sort of tingly and wholly outside of my experience (and I'm an old guy with lots of experience). I also remember giving feedback about the twitching it caused and how odd it felt—it became very pronounced once he was spot-on. After that, he applied the general anesthesia while I was counting backwards from 10 and I don't remember where I stopped, but it was well before I got to 1. ~*~

Once your anesthesiologist locates your nerve, the remainder of the peripheral block placement procedure is similar to the placement of a spinal or epidural; the major difference is the location where the needle is placed. The needle used to inject medication during a peripheral nerve block is relatively small; therefore, your anesthesiologist may or may not numb your skin before the needle is placed. The vast majority of patients who get a peripheral nerve block will also receive medication in their IV to help them relax during the procedure. Some patients have a single dose of medication injected into the nerve, and others have a catheter placed so that pain medication can be continuously infused over time. A single dose of medication can last eight to eighteen hours. A catheter allows you to experience pain relief for as long as the catheter is in place and medication is being given. The same type of medication is used in both central and peripheral anesthetic blocks; however, the doses are different.

Dr. Checa's Recommendations

There are many factors to consider when choosing the anesthetic option that's best for you. Safety will always be the top priority. Assuming that you don't have any significant health concerns that limit your anesthesia options, I've found that most patients choose general anesthesia. While some adventurous folks enjoy experiencing their surgery first hand, most are more comfortable being completely asleep during the entire surgical procedure.

A significant concern for many patients is the fear of waking up from surgery in pain. While intravenous pain medication does a very good job of mitigating much of your postoperative pain, regional anesthesia (combined with going to sleep) may enable you to wake up from your surgery almost completely free of pain. If immediate postoperative pain control is a significant concern for you, I highly recommend discussing the possibility of a regional anesthetic block with your surgeon and anesthesiologist. Almost all anesthesia providers are very familiar—and comfortable with—performing spinal and epidural anesthesia; therefore, these may be your best bet for regional anesthesia. Having an epidural catheter placed is an excellent option for ongoing postoperative pain relief because it can be left in for a day or two after surgery and continues to provide pain relief. However, this may not be an option for you if you're taking high-dose blood thinners to prevent blood clots following your surgery. If you're *not* able to have an epidural catheter placed for medical reasons, I've found that a well-placed spinal block with a long acting pain medication is the best way to maximize your postoperative pain control.

I hope this description of anesthesia options was helpful to you. For many people, the mystery of the process is what causes anxiety. Rest assured that, should you decide to have your hip or knee replaced, there are many anesthesia options available to make the process less painful and less anxiety provoking. Be sure to communicate your expectations and preferences to your surgeon and anesthesiologist prior to surgery. Take comfort in the fact that administration of anesthesia for surgery has evolved into very safe and effective techniques over the years.

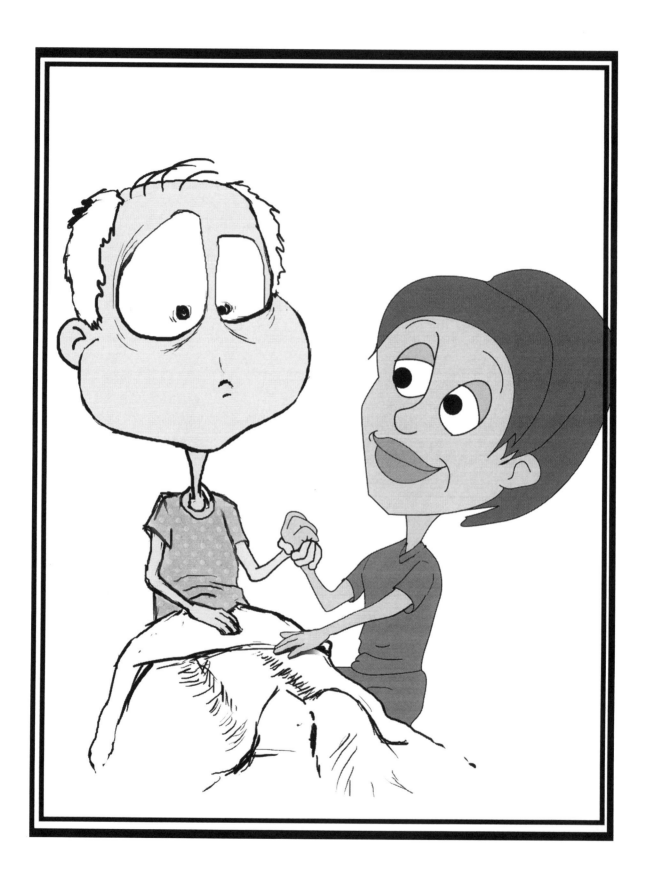

The Day of Surgery

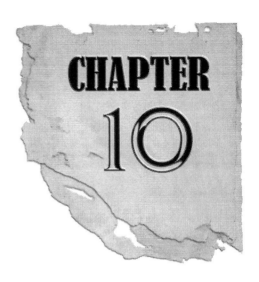

by Dr. Hugate

The day is finally here! You're excited to finally be getting something done about your pain, but at the same time nervous that you're going in for surgery. It's normal to be nervous. Don't be ashamed and don't try to hide it—speak about your concerns with your surgeon. Something else you can do to help make the process more familiar to you and reduce your anxiety is what you're doing right now: arming yourself with knowledge. I have written this chapter, but it includes frequent comments by Robert so we can bring you two perspectives on the same events. This chapter is a step-by-step description of the BIG day—the day of surgery. Keep in mind that while events may vary slightly from institution to institution, this will be a general guide for your journey on the day of surgery.

Preoperative Considerations

It's important to point out a couple of things that can ruin your day. First, it's essential that you arrive for your surgery at the hospital with an empty stomach. Your stomach must be empty because there's a chance that the anesthesiologist may have to put a breathing tube in your throat (a process called "intubation"). This is done routinely when you elect to use general anesthesia, and is a stand-by option if you decide to have any other form of anesthesia. Intubation can sometimes cause one to gag, even if you're asleep during the intubation process and are wholly unaware of the events. If you have a full stomach and gag during the insertion of this tube, you can suffer an event called "aspiration," which occurs when some of the fluid from your stomach gets inhaled into your lungs. This can be a dangerous event that can cause pneumonia and difficulty getting oxygen into your bloodstream. If the stomach is empty when this occurs, there's much less volume of fluid in your stomach and therefore your risk for a significant aspiration event will be much smaller. Either your surgeon's office or your anesthesiologist should instruct you to let you know when you must stop eating and/or drinking before surgery (I typically ask my patients to not eat or drink anything after midnight the night before surgery). Don't forget (or disregard) their instructions: if you arrive for surgery at the hospital with a full stomach, your surgery will be delayed or even cancelled!

Also if you're on medications, please contact the surgeon's office well in advance of surgery and ask them which medications are to be taken and which are not to be taken in the weeks and days before surgery. The same goes for nutritional supplements, vitamins, and all other naturopathic medications. Some people don't think of these as medications and therefore omit them when asked what medications they're on. It's important that your surgeon know what you're taking because naturopathic medications and/or supplements can impart detrimental effects when taken near the time of your surgery and even interact with the medications your surgeon prescribes.

Here are a couple of additional practical tips: whenever possible, schedule your surgery for early in the week. This depends on the institution of course, but some hospitals don't run a full staff on weekends, so you may not get the same level of care that you would during the week. For example, during the weekday you may get a physical therapy session twice a day, whereas on the weekend it may only be once a day. If your surgery is on a Monday or a Tuesday, you will likely be out of the hospital before the weekend, and this won't be an issue.

 Holland's Comment: Also make sure your surgeon isn't leaving town right after your surgery for whatever reason. If she is, reschedule! You will want your surgeon in town for the five to six days following surgery if possible so if there are any problems, she is there for you. ~*~

Another tip: try to have your surgery scheduled as the first one of the day. We surgeons are early risers and there is generally no issue with being "awake enough" to do the surgery. In fact we're at our sharpest early in the day because we have no mental or physical fatigue to deal with. For that reason, if you're able to get your case scheduled as the first case of the day, you'll get your surgeon at her sharpest. This will also give you more time to recover on the day of surgery, and may also buy you an extra session of physical therapy that afternoon, which is good. Although it'll require that you get up very early to be at the hospital for a first-start case, this is time well spent.

Admission and Preparation for Surgery

Your first contact with the hospital on your day of surgery will be when you report to Hospital Admissions to check in for your procedure. This usually happens two to three hours prior to the planned start-time for your surgery. You'll be greeted by a receptionist there who will gather information about you and your insurance. You'll need identification and your insurance card. If you have a living will or medical power of attorney, you'll be asked for it then and it will be placed in your chart. You'll receive an important patient identification bracelet that's to be worn at all times during your hospital stay. It will have a bar code on it that identifies you. This bar code will be used to scan you into the various computers and ensure that your labs, X-rays, and reports are all attributed to the right person. Once you've answered the many questions they have for you in the reception area, you'll be taken back to a surgical holding area. This is where you transform into a patient.

In the surgical holding area, you will be asked to don a "stylish gown." Remember, the opening goes in the back! These gowns are breezy, so you'll be given some warm blankets to cover up and stay warm. The nurse will greet you here and ask you a few more questions. At multiple points during your lead-up to surgery you'll be asked many questions, like:

Who are you?

Who is your surgeon?

What surgery are you having?

Do you have any allergies?

Which side are we operating on?

This is part of a redundant system that helps to significantly reduce the risk of receiving medications you're allergic to and the risk for wrong-site surgery. If your surgeon has ordered any labs, they will be drawn now. An IV will be placed (usually in your arm) to facilitate the administration of fluids and medications.

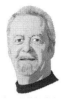

Holland's Comment: I prefer the IV to be about two to three inches above the wrist (in the lower mid-forearm), on the inside of my left arm (because I'm right handed). If nobody can find a vein there, I'll grudgingly allow them to put the IV on the back of my left hand—but having one of these in the back of your hand can be painful.

I prefer not to have the IV in the crook of my arm. If an IV is placed in the crook of your arm, it can make it difficult to bend your arm without pain when you move. With a total joint replacement, you'll be using your arms a great deal to shift yourself about on the bed, so having an IV in the crook of your arm can be uncomfortable.

If the person trying to place the IV can't get it installed after three attempts, simply request that he ask someone else to give it a try. If one person can't set the IV, another one usually can. Sometimes your body will simply not cooperate with a particular staff person and it's not a matter of fault; it just isn't working. The hospital staff will usually ramp the priority up to somebody who is more skilled—sort of an "IV trouble shooter"—if you have a difficult IV to establish. ~*~

You may also be asked at this point to mark the leg and site to be operated on with a skin marker. The nurse will shave the knee or hip to be replaced and they'll scrub the area where the skin incision will be made with an antiseptic cleanser to help reduce the risk of infection. Once you've been prepared to move to the next step in the journey, your nurse will await word from the operating room (OR) that it's time to bring you to the preoperative holding area. If your surgery is the first of the day for your surgeon, you'll likely go to the preoperative area immediately. If yours is not the first surgery of the day, the OR nurse will call to have you transferred to the preoperative holding area when they're near the point of taking you in for surgery.

In the preoperative holding area, you'll be assigned a new nurse and get the same old questions. Again, it's not that the previous nurses weren't paying attention to the answers you gave the first time. There is redundant questioning built into the system to avoid medical mistakes. The nurse here will verify that your labs are complete and make sure that no other testing is necessary before going into surgery. Here you'll meet your surgical team. The nurse will also hang a bag of IV antibiotics on your IV pole to be administered by the anesthesiologist before the surgery begins. Having the antibiotics in your blood stream at the time of incision has been shown to significantly reduce the risk of infection. The anesthesiologist will chat with you briefly and perhaps go over your medical history again. At this time, he'll discuss the type of anesthetic to be used for your operation.

132

You'll also meet the nurse that will be taking care of you in the operating room, and again, more of the same questions. Often the surgical assistant or physician assistant will meet with you here and may do some last minute paperwork. You'll then meet with your surgeon to go over the plan one last time. Your surgeon will sign the hip or knee to be operated on to make sure you're both in agreement.

Ask any remaining questions you may have at this time. Importantly, before you receive any anesthetic medications or sedatives, you and the surgeon will discuss one more time the risks, benefits, and alternatives to performing this operation, and if you are willing, you will sign the consent form. The consent form allows the surgeon to perform your surgery and also demonstrates that you have received the appropriate information needed to consent to the surgery. Once all of this has occurred, your friend or guest will be escorted to the OR waiting room and you'll be given IV medications to help you relax. Then you'll be wheeled to your operating room. What you remember next will depend on how much sedative the anesthesiologist gave you and how sensitive you are to the medications.

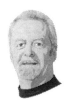

Holland's Comment: I have always found the ride on the gurney to the operating room to be a sort of surreal and dream-like episode. By the time I'm being wheeled about the various corridors leading to the OR, I'm in la-la-land—such is the effect of the tranquilizers Dr. Hugate just mentioned. And before I know it, I'm there!

Then, a team of really friendly people—whom I never remember except for their smiling eyes (as they have their surgical masks on), start talking to me and doing more pre-surgical prep. Next, they move me from the gurney to the operating table—a team effort. For my surgeries, they used the sheet underneath me to help transfer me, lifting as a unit on command. This little caper was lots of fun, probably because by then, I was on cloud nine anyway.

I always take this opportunity to have a joke memorized and ask them if they want to hear it. They always do, and they'll hold off putting you under until you tell them. I have a reason for this—laughter puts the team at ease. It breaks up tension and sets a tone for them throughout the remainder of the surgery. It's well known that laughter is the best medicine. Find a good joke, practice it, and have it memorized for this very special moment. ~*~

The Operating Room

The first thing you'll notice in the operating room is that it's cold. The reason we keep the operating room cold is that cooler temperatures reduce the ability for bacteria to multiply, and therefore the risk of infection is reduced. The next thing you'll notice is that it's bright (for obvious reasons). The surgical scrub tech will be in the room and have all of the instruments laid out on a sterile table ready for your operation. Your gurney will be rolled alongside the operating room table and you'll be asked to scoot over. Sometimes we will help you move over by using a sliding board or a sheet. We typically have patients lie on their backs with their arms out to the side initially. The bed is narrow, so be careful and don't shift around. Once in position, your anesthesiologist will place some monitors on your chest, back and hand. You'll hear a symphony of beeps and bells all indicating that you are alive and well. At this point, if you have elected to have a spinal, epidural, or nerve block anesthetic your anesthesiologist will get that procedure started. At some hospitals you'll have these procedures performed before you go into the OR in a separate room called a "block room" because it's dedicated to performing nerve blocks. Once your anesthetic is ready, you drift off to sleep and the surgery begins. I'll go over the steps in the operation (for those who want to know) in *Chapter 11, The Operations*.

Once the anesthesia starts, you really lose all sense of time. The procedure may take an hour or more, but to you it seems like only a few moments passed. Surgeons often play music to calm their nerves during surgery, so if you hear music, you're not imagining things. You may even (though not likely) remember leaving the OR on a gurney. Some people emerge from anesthesia asking "When are you gonna start, Doc?" The amount of recollection you have really depends on your anesthetic, which was described by Dr. Checa in "Anesthesia Options in Joint Replacement Surgery."

Recovery Room

Your next stop is the recovery room (also called the Post Anesthesia Care Unit or PACU). Here a team of specialized nurses will monitor you while you recover from the anesthesia. Again, depending on what anesthesia you received, this may take a longer or shorter amount of time. These nurses do a great job of keeping you comfortable, making sure any nausea is taken care of, and watching your overall, general well-being. They'll be checking your pulse and nerve function as you recover as well.

If you had your knee replaced, your knee may be placed in a machine that gently moves it back and forth called a CPM (continuous passive motion) machine. This helps to get your knee motion back right out of the gate. You'll have a large dressing on your wound, consisting of some combination of gauze, absorbent pads, and tape or compressive dressing like ACE wrap (aka ACE Elastic Bandage). Your surgeon may place a drain as well. A drain is a small plastic tube that goes through your skin and into the area where your surgeon has just placed the new joint implant. The purpose of the drain is to evacuate any blood that may be accumulating inside your wound so that you don't fill your wound with blood. Having a large amount of blood accumulate in the wound would make it difficult for you to move the joint after surgery.

You'll be in the recovery room for approximately two hours if all goes well. Once you have recovered sufficiently from surgery, your PACU nurse will call the floor and transfer you to your room so that you may begin the journey of healing, recovery, and rehabilitation.

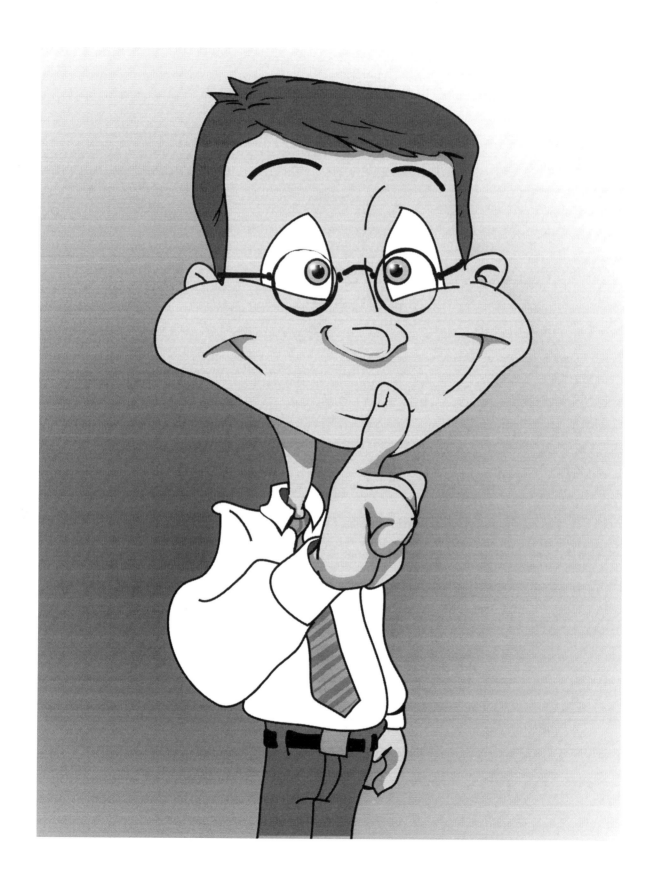

The Operations

CHAPTER 11

by Dr. Hugate

This is the chapter of our handbook in which I let you in on all of my *secrets*. What goes on after you're asleep in the operating room? For some, they prefer not to know the details of the surgery and I can certainly respect this. If this is the case with you, I would urge you to stop reading this chapter and move on to the next. If, however, you're one of those folks who likes to know what goes on "behind the scenes," then read on. I'll give you as much detail as you need, but I'll try not to go overboard. I don't want you to drown in technicalities, and if I tell you all my tricks, you may try this on your own! So, we'll stick with the major points and I'll throw in some illustrations along the way as I describe the procedures.

I'll start with a description of the "pre-surgical routine," which is common to both types of surgery, and then move on to the specifics of either hip or knee replacement surgery itself. Again, all of what I am about to describe happens after the patient is either sedated or asleep in the operating room.

Presurgical Routine

There is a presurgery checklist that all surgeons go through in their mind before operating, like the preflight checklist that your pilot performs before takeoff. Mine begins with re-verifying the surgical site, which was marked with my initials in the preoperative area using a permanent marker. This may seem like a trivial thing, but to this day (on rare occasions) there are reports of surgeons operating on the wrong extremity. This system has served me well.

Once the patient is in the operating room (OR), I always confirm that the anesthesiologist has started the antibiotic drip before we start the surgery. Studies have shown that when the antibiotics are in your bloodstream prior to surgery, the risk of infection is reduced. At this time, we also do what's referred to as a "time out." Everyone in the OR stops what they're doing to hear the lead nurse in the OR make a statement about the procedure. The nurse will verbally verify the patient's name, date of birth, medical record number, and medical allergies, and will confirm that the joint replacement parts are in the room. They confirm that the antibiotics have been given and also state the position of the patient, the intended procedure, and the correct extremity as evidenced by the patient's verbal report, the consent form, and the surgeon's initials placed on the operative side... whew! All of this must be done routinely to ensure that no mistakes are made. The nurse may place a Foley catheter (a catheter placed into the bladder to collect urine) depending on what type of anesthesia was given. If a spinal or epidural anesthetic is given we typically employ a Foley catheter. I will often put the X-rays up in the room to use as a guide.

We also verify that the *laminar air flow* is on. This is a type of specialized air flow built in to the OR that reduces the amount of bacteria being swept up from the floor and into the air. The surgical team (surgeon, assistant, and scrub tech—described in **Chapter 7, Your Medical Team** of this handbook) will then have a brief discussion about the plan on this particular case.

Next, I direct one of my assistants to tape the outer door of the OR shut and put up a sign indicating "No Entry Allowed!" The reason for this is that studies have shown that the more traffic in the OR (people coming in and out), the higher the risk for infection. There's another door that's open to those who need to come in, but it opens from a sterile corridor and therefore is much less likely to cause bacteria to enter the room.

Now, we "position" the patient for the surgery. The critical process of positioning a patient serves two purposes. First, it puts the patient's hip or knee in the correct orientation so the surgeon can appropriately expose the joint, prepare the bones, and align the components of the joint replacement. The second purpose of positioning is to avoid pressure sores or pressure injury to nerves.

Being in surgery is not exactly like going for a nap from the patient's perspective. When you and I sleep, we are constantly moving around. Why is that? Because after a few minutes the areas of our body with the highest contact pressure on the bed become sore and our brain tells us to shift around a bit to avoid pain and injury to that area. When a patient has surgery, she doesn't have the luxury of shifting around. She's in the same position until the surgery is done, whether it's a one-hour or ten-hour-long surgery. One of the dangers is if there's excess pressure on any particular body part, you could easily develop either a pressure ulcer or even nerve damage.

Therefore, we're very careful to place the patient in a position such that the pressure of the OR table is evenly distributed and all areas near major nerves are especially padded or relieved of pressure. Now let's move on to the individual procedure descriptions.

Knee Replacement

For knee replacement surgery, the next thing we do is put the patient and her leg in the correct position and prepare the leg. I will often put a small roll of towels under the buttock to help turn the leg inwards a bit. Normally our legs rotate outwardly when we lay down such that the toes are pointing off to the side at an angle. I like to put enough rolls under the buttock so that the toe is pointing straight up. This helps me align the components during the surgery. We will also place a tourniquet on the thigh at this time. The tourniquet is an inflatable cuff that goes around the thigh just below the hip and is connected to an air pump. When inflated, it allows us to block blood from flowing into the leg and knee during surgery. This makes for less blood loss and helps the surgeon visualize things better as well.

Preparing For Surgery

At this point, my assistant and I go off to the sink and begin to aseptically scrub our hands and forearms. While we are scrubbing up, the OR nurse begins the same process (of aseptic scrubbing) on the knee and leg to be operated on. The nurse typically takes about ten minutes to wash the knee and leg. This allows enough contact time for the sterilizing agents to kill the bacteria on the skin.

Once my assistant and I have scrubbed our hands, we enter the operating room and receive our helmets, gowns, and gloves from the scrub tech. This is done in such a manner as to keep everything sterile. In the OR I use a "space suit," which is an enclosed, ventilated helmet so that no flakes of skin or hair from the surgical team will fall into the wound and cause infection.

At this point we begin a process called "draping". Draping is the placement of sterile drapes over the patient so only the body part we're operating on is exposed. If done properly, there are at least two layers of drapes over any unsterile surface. This redundancy ensures that if the outer drape tears, there is still a layer of protection below. Once the drapes are in place, everyone takes their places.

The scrub tech, surgeon, and assistant all have positions that they routinely occupy for the procedure. We adjust the lights in the OR such that they're pointing directly at the knee from many different angles. At this point I ask the anesthesiologist if the patient is ready for me to begin the procedure. With the big, "OK!" we then begin.

First we elevate the leg to allow most of the blood to drain out and then inflate the tourniquet. The tourniquet is monitored by the anesthesiologist and the nurse to ensure that it's at the right pressure and to make certain it doesn't stay on the leg too long. Once the tourniquet is inflated, I make the incision.

Performing the Knee Replacement Surgery

The knee incision I use runs over the front of the knee, curved slightly toward the inside of the kneecap. It's made just long enough for me to see what I have to do and insert the knee implant safely. For me that's about six inches of incision in an average-sized person. Once the incision is made, I use a device called an "electro-cautery" to dissect through the tissues. It uses electricity to burn the tissue and results in less blood loss because it seals the small blood vessels as it goes.

After the incision, we continue straight down until we get to the patella (kneecap), patellar ligament, and the quadriceps muscles called the "extensor mechanism." This large group of muscles in front of the thigh are responsible for straightening the knee. Once we get to this layer we have to make another incision along the inside of the *extensor mechanism* to get to the knee joint. Here we encounter joint fluid (aka synovial fluid) and this is removed with a suction device. We then release the tissues along the inside of the tibia (the lower leg bone) and bend the knee to expose the surfaces of the knee joint. We also "flip" the kneecap over at this point to get it out of the way and allow us to work on the knee surfaces safely.

With the knee bent and the patella flipped out of the way, I usually start on the femoral side (thigh bone) of the knee joint. The first thing we do here is remove the cruciate ligaments. Next, we drill a hole in the end of the femur bone and place a long rod into the canal. This allows me a point of reference. Remember that many knees with severe arthritis are so worn they've become deformed. Because of this, part of the knee replacement process is not only giving you new, pain-free joint surfaces, but also re-aligning them so your knee is no longer deformed (bowlegged or knock-kneed). With this in mind we surgeons know the exact angle that the joint should make with the femur and use a special cutting guide to remove the very end of the femur at the angle that is appropriate.

Because every person's anatomy is somewhat unique, at this point in the operation we use a special jig to determine the appropriate size implant for the individual. The implant components themselves are identical in function but come as sets in a variety of matched sizes (**See Figure 11.1**). Once the correct size is determined, we select from a set of differentially sized cutting jigs that are then mounted through the use of pins. A specialized, surgical, oscillating bone-saw is used to make the proper bone cuts and, once the cuts have been made, there is a "trial" implant that can be impacted onto the bone to ensure the cuts were made properly.

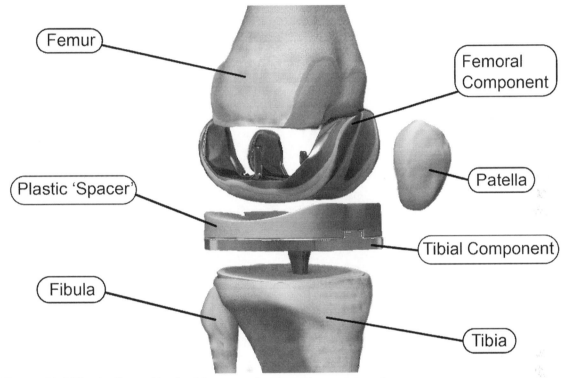

Figure 11.1 Illustration of typical knee replacement components

Now, we move on to the tibia (the lower leg bone). My assistant places retractors such that the entire tibial plateau (top of the lower leg bone) is visible. We remove what's left of the meniscus cartilage, place an external alignment guide that starts at the ankle and allows us to put the tibial component perpendicular to the axis of the tibia like the cross on the letter "T" (again, this is done to correct any deformity). We then use a small cutting guide to make the cut. We cut just enough of the bone away so that the replacement pieces fit snugly. Once the bone is cut away, we select the appropriate size for the implant and place a trial implant into position. If it covers and fills the bone surface properly, then we select that size and make a few additional preparations to the tibia. We use your own anatomy to help determine the proper rotational alignment of the implant. At this point, the knee cap is flipped back over and sized, then a flat cut is made on the back surface to receive the trial patella component (a small plastic "button"). Using another guide, small peg holes are drilled to match those on the patellar component implant and the trial component is placed into position.

Once the femur, tibia, and patella have been prepared, with all three of these trial pieces in place, we begin assessing how they fit *together*. We usually start with about a 10mm plastic trial spacer in between the components. With this spacer in place we range the knee (bending and straightening) through its entire motion. Does it come fully straight? If not the plastic spacer may be too big. Does it bend fully? If not the femur component may be too big. Does the patella stay in its "groove" during motion? If not the rotation of one or both components may be off. We also try to bend the knee from side to side to see if we have sized the components properly. A normal knee does not bend (much) from side to side and through years of experience, surgeons get a feel for how much is enough to make it stable but not too tight. If the knee fails any of these tests, there are a prescribed number of adjustments that need to be made. The knee is then re-trialed until I am satisfied with the outcome.

When all of the trials fit well and the knee motion and stability have been verified, the brand new knee parts are opened and placed on the sterile back table. These are the actual pieces that will be implanted. The only part we don't open yet is the plastic spacer—called the "poly." The components are touched by personnel as little as possible to avoid contamination. At this point, my scrub tech will begin mixing the methyl methacrylate. This is a type of two-part cement that's used to stick the components on to the bone. My surgical assistant then uses a powerful "water jet" device to clean the surfaces of the bone so the cement will help the implant components stick to the bone better. This is another good reason to have a tourniquet. The tourniquet prevents bleeding of the bone surfaces and allows us to get a dry surface to cement the parts onto. If the tourniquet were down, the bone channels would bleed, wetting the end of the bone, and the cement wouldn't adhere to the bone appropriately. If my patient is at higher risk for infection, then I will have my scrub tech add antibiotics to the methyl methacrylate cement as well. Once the mixture is ready, we then cement the new implant parts into position. It takes about ten minutes for the cement to cure, so during that time I compress the parts against the bone and remove any excess material.

Once the cement sets, we range the knee through motion again with a trial spacer in place to ensure that it's still acceptable. Once verified, the real "poly spacer" component is opened and inserted into place (this piece actually locks mechanically into place). We double check again to see that there is no extra cement material hanging around, and if so, we remove it. We then start the process of closing the wound.

Remember, there is little or no bleeding up to this point because the tourniquet is inflated. We do, however, anticipate some bleeding will occur after the tourniquet is deflated (let down). For that reason, some surgeons now place a small plastic tube (drain) into the wound through the skin above your knee to allow any blood which will accumulate to be evacuated for the day or two after surgery. With the drain in place, we now begin closing the wound in layers. Just prior to closure, the scrub tech and the nurse will count the needles and the sponges used during the operation to ensure that none were left in the wound. This is done twice prior to concluding the operation.

We then wash out the wound with saline and begin the process of closing the wound. The first layer of closure is the extensor mechanism (remember the big tendon in the front of the knee?). This is closed from top to bottom with large sutures, as it takes most of the stress when the knee is bent after surgery. After the inner sutures are all placed, we then bend the knee back and forth to ensure these are strong enough to withstand range of motion. Next we put another layer of sutures just under the skin layer to bring the skin edges together. These sutures are absorbable (meaning they will disappear a few months after the surgery). The final layer of sutures is the external skin layer. Surgeons vary in preference but I tend to use either surgical clips or nylon sutures to close this layer. Again, there can be a lot of tension on this skin when you bend your knee after knee replacement and these types of skin closures are very rugged and strong. The last thing we want is for your incision to pop open while bending your knee.

Now that the skin is closed we place a sterile dressing on the knee consisting of a no-stick petroleum gauze, regular gauze, and absorbent pads encircled by a compressive ACE Wrap to keep the swelling to a minimum. The tourniquet is let down and suction is applied to the drain tube. The anesthesiologist awakens the patient and they're off to the recovery room.

Hip Replacement

Before we talk about the positioning of a patient for hip replacement surgery, I need to explain some things about the various, different "approaches" used in hip replacement surgery. An "approach" is surgical jargon for the path that we take to get to the hip joint. The *approach* helps describe where the incision is and, more importantly, what muscles are affected during the surgery. In the hip, one can perform an "anterior" approach (incision is in front of the hip), lateral approach (incision across the top of the mound formed by the hipbone) or a posterior approach (incision over the buttock). There are other approaches, but these are the main ones. Each approach has different advantages and disadvantages.

For purposes of this handbook, I'll describe the way I perform hip replacement. I tend to use the posterior approach for most of the hip replacements I perform. The incision starts on the outer aspect of the hip and is curved back along the buttock. I use this approach for a few reasons. First, it avoids damage to the important muscles around the hip, which allows for less limp and faster recovery after surgery. Second, this approach can be done through a fairly small incision. Also, this approach allows us to have the major nerve (called the sciatic nerve) in direct view during the surgery... which allows me to know where it is at all times and therefore avoid injuring it.

With that said, for the posterior approach, I position the patient on his side with the operative hip up. We use special, padded clamps to hold the patient in position so he doesn't shift around or fall off the operating table during the surgery. Having the patient in a fixed position also is very helpful for ensuring that the hip replacement parts are aligned correctly. A pillow is placed between the arms, and the legs are padded and slightly bent at the knee to avoid stretching or injuring the nerves.

With the patient in this position, I feel where the heels line up to get a sense of what their correct leg length should be. Unlike in knee replacement surgery, in hip replacement surgery one of the common complications is that the leg is not restored to the proper length. This is just one of the steps I use to help ensure that the leg lengths will end up being correct. Later with the hip replacement in place, I will compare how the heels line up again and compare it to how they lined up at the beginning of surgery.

Once the patient is properly positioned and well padded, my assistant and I go off to the scrub sink. The process of scrubbing our hands, preparing the patient's skin, donning the operative gowns, and draping the patient are all similar to that which occurred during my description of the knee replacement earlier—so I'll skip that description here. At this point, I ask the anesthesiologist if the patient is ready for me to begin the procedure. When I get the thumbs up, we begin.

Performing the Hip Replacement Surgery

The incision is the next step. A curved incision is made starting on the outer aspect of the hip and curving around the back in the buttocks. For an average sized individual, this incision is approximately 5" in length. It can be longer or shorter depending on how big the patient is. We then work our way down to the muscles.

The first muscle we encounter is the famous gluteus maximus muscle. This is the muscle that makes up the majority of the buttock. We must get through this muscle to get to the back of the hip joint. It's important to realize that we don't release or cut across this muscle. It stays entirely intact through the operation. Muscles have layers of parallel fibers running in the same direction. It's therefore possible to open a "window" in the muscle that can later be closed rather than cutting across the fibers of the muscle and destroying it. Remember the function of the muscles is important for avoiding a limp and speeding your recovery.

Once we make the window in the gluteus maximus muscle we now see several structures. There is usually a thin layer of fat here which is then folded back. Under the fat is a small muscle called the piriformis muscle. This is the first in a series of small muscles behind the hip called _short external rotators_. The piriformis muscle is released from the hipbone where it attaches and is later repaired at the end of the procedure. This is a small

144

muscle (about the size of your thumb). Behind the piriformis muscle is the large and very important sciatic nerve. We take careful note of where it is as this helps avoid injury to this nerve going forward.

With the piriformis muscle out of the way, we're now looking at the back of the hip capsule. The hip (like the knee) has a large thick capsule surrounding it to help contain the lubricating joint fluid and help prevent the hip from dislocating. The back half of the capsule is removed to reveal the ball-and-socket hip joint. My assistant then turns the leg and pulls in such a way as to dislocate the hip ("pop" it out of joint). This allows us to separate the ball from the socket and work on each one individually. Next, we use our preoperative X-rays to help decide where to make our cut on the neck of the femur. With an oscillating bone saw, we then remove the old worn out ball from the hip.

Once the ball is out of the way, I start on preparing the new cup. We place retractors so that I can see down into the cup and the area surrounding it. Sometimes the arthritis is so bad that the ball or socket are no longer round, so the goal at this point in the operation is to remove the arthritic joint surface and make a nice round hemispherical cup to accept your hip replacement parts. We use a series of spherical reamers. These look like cheese-graters. They're placed in your original cup and rotated under power (using a power reamer). As we go up in size, we remove more of the old arthritic joint surface. Eventually we are left with a perfectly hemispherical space ready for your new prosthetic cup. The new cup is then impacted into position with a press fit. Remember, this is a metal shell and we will later be placing a "liner" in that shell to act as the bearing surface of your ball and socket joint. The position of the cup is critical, because it affects your stability (that is, how hard it is for you to dislocate this new hip after surgery). Once the cup is in place, I usually place one screw through the cup into the bone to make sure it's stable and solid. With the new cup in place, we then go on to replacing the "ball" part of the joint on the femur where we cut the original, arthritic ball off.

The top of the femur is now brought up and into view by my assistant. The femur, like all long bones, is much like a pipe. The hard, outer surface provides the strength and there is softer bone on the inside where the bone marrow resides. The anchor for the ball is a stem that either press fits (or is cemented) into the bone. Therefore, the first step here is to create a path for that stem. We start with a power reamer to clean out the contents from the center of the bone and create this path. This is also where we can determine what the appropriate size for the implant is. We then place a series of "broaches" into the bone. Broaches are like rasps shaped in the size of the stem that we will eventually use. The broaches start small and get bigger until we get a tight fit. Again, this clears the way for the stem and helps us choose the correct size.

With the appropriate-sized broach in the bone we now are able to "trial" the hip. This is critical to getting the leg lengths correct and making the hip stable enough that it won't dislocate after the surgery is done. Essentially, we put the ball back into the socket. We can feel the leg lengths at this point or even take an X-ray to ensure that the leg lengths

145

are equal if necessary. We also move the hip around to see how difficult it is to dislocate. If it dislocates easily, we can do a number of things: either change the position of the cup, change the position of the stem, or change the ball. The balls come in longer or shorter arrangements and also larger and smaller diameters. Once we have positioned everything optimally and chosen the appropriate sizes, we then remove all of the trial components and place the real implants. The hip is re-examined now with the real components in place to ensure that the hip is stable and leg lengths are equal.

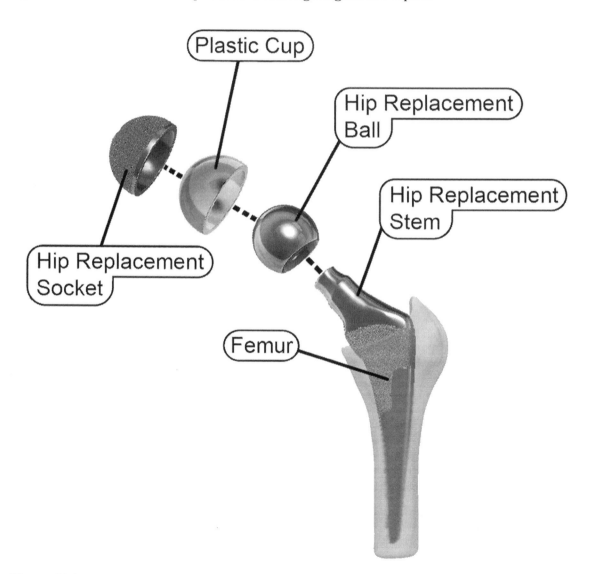

Figure 11.2 Illustration of typical hip replacement components

We then wash out the wound with saline and begin the process of closing. A drain is placed within the wound and taken out through the skin above the incision. The purpose of the drain is to evacuate any blood that may accumulate within the wound after surgery and is typically removed a day or two after the surgery. The piriformis tendon is repaired back to its original location with sutures. The gluteus maximus window is closed and the skin is then closed. I tend to use absorbable sutures (that dissolve away in a few months) for hip replacements. These are placed all under the skin so that they do not have to be removed. We then place small adherent paper strips over the incision to provide support and place a dressing over the hip comprised of no-stick petroleum gauze, plain gauze, absorbent pads, and tape. The anesthesiologist awakens the patient and the two of them are off to the recovery room.

Of course there are variations on what I have described. Every surgeon does things slightly differently—different approach, different position, different order, etc.—but all of the major processes are the same. These are my systems for a routine knee and hip replacement…a brief down-and-dirty look at the processes we surgeons take you through in the OR. I hope this chapter was informative and helps to take some of the mystery out of the process for you.

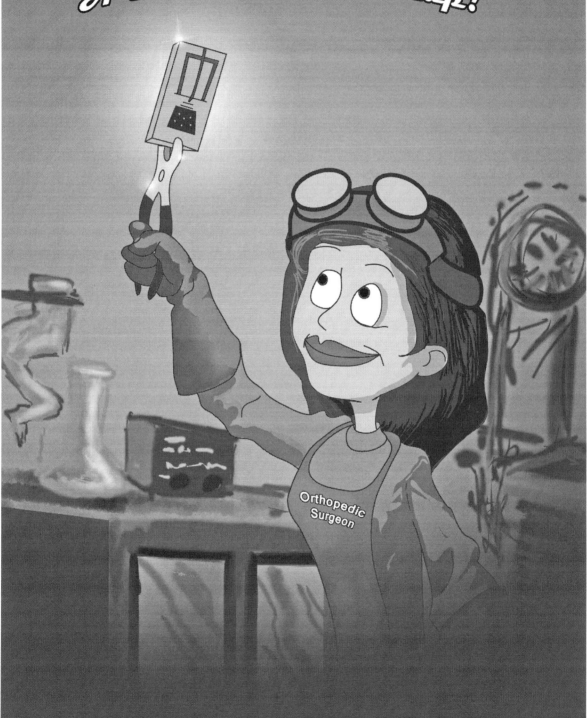

Methods, Types, and Designs of Joint Replacements

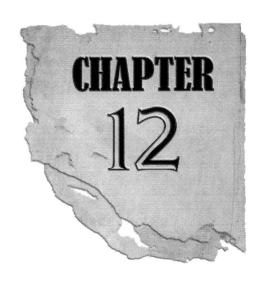

CHAPTER 12

by Dr. Hugate

Hip and knee replacements come in many different flavors and varieties. The standard hip and knee replacement operations have been in mainstream use since the 1970s. These procedures have improved function and reduced pain for millions of patients since their inception. About 95 percent of people receiving hip or knee replacements report good to excellent results without major complications. Studies which look at the effectiveness of surgery consistently rank joint replacement as among the most successful surgeries performed. Still, there is always room for improvement and, as such, each successive generation of orthopedic surgeons has done what we are supposed to do: attempt to "build a better mouse trap!" In this chapter we'll discuss a few of the different variations of hip and knee replacement procedures, modern evolutions of the implants, and the surgical techniques used to install these implants.

Durability Issues

In addition to our own efforts as surgeons to improve implants and surgical techniques, the public is demanding improved implants as well. Each year, patients considering joint replacement get younger and younger. In the early days, hip and knee replacement were considered options only for *low-demand*, 70-year-old and older patients with severe arthritis. By low-demand, I mean patients who are not very active- do not participate in impact activities, running, contact sports, and so on. Accordingly, with excellent results in these low-demand populations, and as time has passed, the age group of patients considering joint replacements has steadily crept downwards. Nowadays it's more common for someone in their 60s or even 50s to undergo joint replacement, and for a variety of reasons.

Why is the age of the patient even an issue? Remember that joint replacements consist of *mechanical,* not biological parts. They can't regenerate or repair themselves when injured like most biological tissues can. This means the parts of a joint replacement can wear out over time. Consider that if you receive a joint replacement at age 70 and are fairly low demand, the replacement will probably last you the rest of your life. Now consider if I put that same joint replacement in an active 50 year old. The average 50 year old is heavier than the average 70 year old, which increases the stress on the joint replacement significantly. The 50 year old probably engages in more activity than the average 70 year old, and this too increases stress on the new joint. The 50 year old also has (on average) about another twenty-five years to live, which further increases the stresses on the joint over the implant's lifetime. Do you see the pattern here?

There's an analogy I like to use in my office because it helps my patients understand this concept. Consider the tires on a car. Suppose you have two cars, and each of those two cars gets a brand new set of tires. Which set of tires will wear out first? In general, the tires on the heavier car, that is driven more often, and driven more *aggressively* (and at higher speeds), will be the set of tires to wear out first, right? On the lighter car, which is driven below the speed limit and only a few miles per week, the tires would last many years. The same holds true for joint replacements: the less you weigh and the less active you are, the longer your joint replacement will last before wearing out.

All this can add up to problems with the joint replacement when performed on younger patients. In our example, the 50-year-old patient will likely have to undergo another one (or two) operations through the course of his lifetime to replace or repair worn out parts of the joint replacement. This is why orthopedic surgeons, as a group, make a concerted effort to avoid replacing joints in younger people if at all possible. This includes the use of all forms of alternative treatments as mentioned in **Chapter 1, When Do You "Need" a Joint Replacement?**.

With these factors in mind, one of the major questions which drives the evolution of total joint replacement technology is, "How can we change the techniques and/or implants in joint replacement surgery such that people can be more active—for a longer period of time—without their joint replacement wearing out?" This is the million-dollar question. If we can answer this question well enough, it opens the door to joint replacement for younger patients who may be suffering just as badly as their older counterparts but have not had a great surgical option up to this point.

To address these issues, surgeons and engineers have employed a number of strategies, mainly focusing on the materials used in the joint replacement. The parts that generally wear out are the *bearing surfaces*. Remember, bearing surfaces are a part of any mechanical

150

system where two parts rub together. In a hip replacement, the bearing surfaces are located where the ball and socket come together. In a knee replacement the bearing surface is where the metal components rub against the plastic spacer. In either case, over the lifetime of an implant, these two surfaces can rub against one another for millions of cycles. Every time a step is taken, these parts rub together. Therefore, the goal is to reduce the friction at these bearing surfaces and reduce how much they wear over a given period of time.

Is Newer Really Better?

Remember as you read about these proposed advances in techniques and implants that *newer* is not always *better*. One of the great difficulties in making new and improved implants is that it takes a long time to know whether a new design is a winner or a stinker. We have mentioned that the average joint replacement lasts about fifteen years. Well, here is the difficulty: suppose Dr. Hotshot designs a new hip replacement system—cutting edge technology and materials with a well-thought-out design. If she starts using that hip replacement for her patients today, it will be about fifteen years before she can fairly compare how her technology stacks up against the "old" technology (which has already been around for fifteen years). Sure, we can take "snapshots" of how the new hip replacement design is performing along the way. If this new hip replacement fails at an unusually high rate, we can assume that it's a bad design and stop using it. But nobody can predict how well a new hip replacement will be doing in fifteen years. For that reason, we must make assumptions, and they aren't always correct. The reason I make you aware of this is so that you don't fall into the "newer is better" school of thought. If I were to have my hip replaced today, I would go with one of the time-proven implants that has been around for years! With that in mind, let's look at some newer technologies, techniques, and trends in hip and knee replacement.

Minimally-invasive Surgery

In addition to design changes of the implants themselves, we surgeons have been busy trying to find better ways to surgically install them. One focus has lately been on length of incision needed (so-called *minimally-invasive surgery*) and how we "approach" the joint during surgery.

First, let's talk about length of incisions. There is no question that the instrumentation used to insert hip and knee replacements has improved, and new techniques have evolved to enable orthopedic surgeons to implant the same joint replacements through smaller incisions. The goal, of course, is to limit the invasiveness of the surgical procedure so that patients have less pain and are able to recover faster and more easily. Over the last decade or so, most surgeons have been well trained in the use of these less invasive techniques for installing hips and knees.

There is a balance that we must strike when surgically installing joint replacements, though. The balance is between minimal invasiveness and our ability to perform the operation safely and consistently. The smaller the incision the more limited is the visibility during the surgical approach. The less your surgeon can see, the greater the struggle for the surgeon and the greater the potential for complications.

Let's use an analogy to help illustrate. Suppose a clever local car mechanic comes up with a way to change the sparkplugs in your car without ever opening the hood. Must be better, right? I mean, wow, that sounds like a magic trick! He's developed a set of tools that snakes through the fender-well of your car and *Poof!* Your spark plugs are swapped out and as good as new. It takes a bit more time than the standard technique, and it is more technically demanding, of course. Your mechanic will need to have the special equipment, and special training, and his technique may cost a bit more—but if he has all of this, you can get your spark plugs changed without even opening the hood. Oh yes, before I forget, the rate of having the spark plugs installed incorrectly is only slightly higher with this technique. The mechanic can't see the spark plugs as he's installing them, so he has to rely on the instruments and his "feel" to get some of the job done correctly... but did I mention that he didn't even have to open the hood?

The first question we all should ask is ourselves is, "Why wouldn't the mechanic just open the hood and change the sparkplugs in the usual way?" I mean this new technique takes more time, costs more, and the complication rate is higher. Here are the questions we should all be asking whenever a revolutionary new technique comes along: "Is there an advantage to not opening the hood and seeing the sparkplugs as the mechanic removes and reinstalls them? Has this mechanic "built a better mousetrap"? Is the car or the driver better off in the long run for his having used this new technique for changing the spark plugs?" Too often new techniques are used as advertisement ploys without facing and answering these critical questions.

Don't get me wrong, I use much smaller incisions than my predecessors did for their hip and knee replacement procedures. My average hip replacement incision is about five inches and knee replacement incision is about six inches long. This is an average, and can be a bit bigger or smaller depending on the size of the patient. This incision is big enough for me to see what I'm doing and no bigger. I have never once heard a patient complain about the length of their five- or six-inch incisions. And yet some surgeons still push for even smaller incisions. Sure, I could perform a knee replacement through a five-inch incision, but it would be a struggle, and the complication rate will inevitably go up—not worth the one-inch reduction in incision length. Here is my plea to any surgeon who may ever replace *my* joints in the future: "Please doctor, use an incision long enough for you to see what you are doing. I would rather you have enough visibility to get the job done right the first time, every time!"

Different Approaches to a Joint

Aside from the *length* of the incision, surgeons are also constantly looking at new and different methods of installing the joints; that is, different *approaches*. The idea is to do as little damage to surrounding tissues as possible while we make our way through the tendons and muscles of your hip or knee during surgery. I most commonly use the "para-patellar" approach to enter the knee joint and enter the hip through the "posterior" approach. These are the most commonly used approaches today because orthopedic surgeons can reliably and consistently perform the operations while doing very little collateral damage. There are other ways in which you can enter the hip and knee joints, however, and surgeons are exploring which routes of entry leave patients with the best outcomes.

While most surgeons are trained in the use of several different approaches to the hip and knee, there are special situations in which different approaches are required. For example, if I perform a hip replacement on a patient who has a spastic muscle condition such as Parkinson's disease, I will use a special approach geared toward reducing the risk of the hip popping out of joint (because the patient may not have good muscular control). The special approach I use may not be the best approach for regaining strength, or eliminating a limp, but is designed to reduce the risk of dislocation. In this case, I'm tailoring the strengths of the approach to the needs of the patient. There are other examples I could cite, but I think you get the overall picture and getting into a technical discussion about the pros and cons of each approach to the hip and knee is beyond the scope of this handbook.

The take-home message is this: your surgeon has trained on and is comfortable performing the approaches they use. I do not think you should select a surgeon based on what approach they use because there is not, in my opinion, a clear advantage of any modern approach to the hip or knee over another (unless there are special circumstances as we've discussed). There are excellent surgeons that use the posterior approach, and the anterior approach, and so on. Most joint replacement surgeons keep abreast of new developments in this complex field of joint replacement surgery. Consequently, if a new technique or approach ever emerges as clearly and significantly superior to the mainstream approaches commonly used today, then surgeons will likely abandon their current techniques and switch to the superior approach. Until then, we will keep using the approaches that we know work well for our patients.

Computer-Guided Joint Replacement

Another newer technology used to help improve the installation of joint replacements is "computer guided" technology. One of the many factors that makes a joint replacement successful is the ability to align the parts correctly. Hip and knee replacement parts should be installed at a prescribed set of angles allowing the force of your weight to cross uniformly through the implant, evenly distributing the load. If the parts are misaligned during installation, the joint may wear out prematurely, perhaps loosen, and may even affect the way you walk (your gait). Also consider the issue of leg length after joint replacement. If the hip joint is not replaced to the correct height, one of your legs will be longer (or shorter) than the other after surgery. The current standard of technology uses a series of guides described in *Chapter 11, The Operations* which allow for the implant to be placed and aligned properly based on the patient's anatomy as seen with preoperative X-rays and discovered more precisely during surgery.

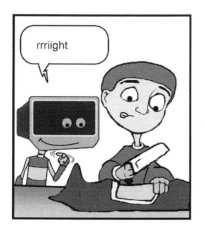 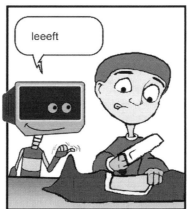 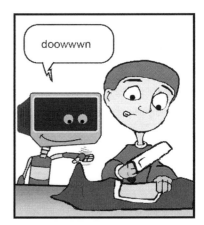

Figure 12.1 Cartoon "OK Doc, a little to the right. No, too far—back to the left—that's it. Now down a little. You've got it!"

Computer-guided technology is currently being explored as a possible way to ensure that the alignment of joints is better and more consistent. The idea is a simple one: the surgeon gets either a CT scan or an MRI of your hip or knee, and that information is fed into a computer. The computer then calculates where the bone cuts should be made in order for your knee or hip to be properly aligned. At the time of surgery, your surgeon places pins in your bone with reflective markers on the ends of the pins. A computerized "eye" in the operating room then senses the position of those reflective markers, and combines this with the information from the aforementioned CT scan or MRI to tell the surgeon where to make the bone cuts. This system has been found to help some surgeons align their patients' joint replacement parts properly. It is not clear if surgeons who do a higher volume of joint replacements are helped significantly with these systems. This technology is evolving and may eventually be more widely used. For now, I believe that surgeons who perform fifty or more hip or knee replacements in a year probably do not benefit from using the computerized systems. As with all things, however, surgeons will continue to watch this technology and it may become more widely used in the future—providing it proves to be helpful in the long run.

Hip Replacement Variations

As we discussed earlier, one of the main focuses in implant design is that of improving longevity of the implant through the use of improved bearing materials that wear less. Many material combinations have been tried for the ball and socket of hip replacements, but in the recent past, the most common materials used as bearing surfaces were a metal (cobalt-chromium steel) ball in a plastic socket (a special plastic called "ultra-high molecular weight polyethylene" or UHMW). The plastic is sometimes referred to as "poly" for short. This gave an excellent, low-friction, low-wear combination that worked well for millions. They did wear out over time, however, and the plastic residue particles that were produced from years of rubbing also created a reaction in the body which caused some of the bone to be dissolved. Some implants even loosened over time. As a result, we are seeing waves of patients today whose hips have not only worn out, but they've lost some of their supportive bone as result of this plastic particle bone-loss reaction. This can be a difficult problem for patients and surgeons alike.

To help reduce or eliminate this issue, surgeons, engineers, and material specialists have worked to improve the wear characteristics of the plastic. There is a process that the plastics undergo during manufacturing called "cross-linking." Without becoming too technical here, the cross-linking of the plastics helps the molecules in the material stick together better, making them less likely to wear and shed the offending plastic particles.

The problem is that the cross-linking process also tends to make the plastic more brittle. Therefore, the trick is to strike a balance between how much cross-linking is necessary to reduce the wear, without making the material too brittle. Also, sterilization of the plastic is now done in an oxygen-free environment to help reduce oxidation of the plastic. Some companies have even started impregnating the plastics with anti-oxidants, like Vitamin E. Suffice it to say there are many techniques being employed to make the plastics constantly better. The newer plastics, because of the additional cross-linking, are referred to as "highly cross-linked poly." Surgeons will typically use this type of plastic socket in patients who are heavier, younger, and who participate in higher demand activities. Of course, it is a bit more expensive than standard plastic sockets, but in my opinion it is worth every penny in these higher-demand patients.

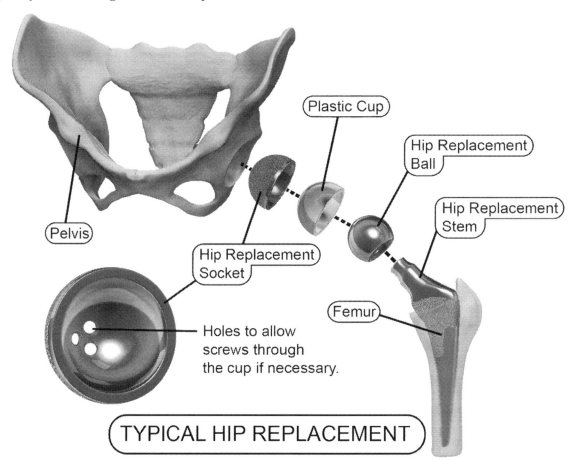

Figure 12.2 Illustration of typical hip replacement hardware components in relationship to the pelvis

There are other materials available as bearing surfaces in hip replacements, and these have become more popular over the years as well. Ceramics are popular for a few reasons. Ceramics are very wear resistant and, because of their material properties, can be

156

manufactured with smoother surfaces, reducing friction. Ceramics can be brittle, however, and there were even a few ceramic hip replacements in the 1990s that cracked and had to be revised. Since that time, advancements in material engineering of these ceramics has virtually eliminated the issue of ceramics cracking. Another issue seen with ceramics lately is the so-called "squeaking" hip. This occurred in a small percentage of patients who received ceramic-on-ceramic hip replacements (meaning both the ball and the socket were made of ceramics). The squeaking was so annoying for some of these patients they actually had the parts swapped out to get rid of the noise! After going through these growing pains, however, ceramics have emerged as an excellent option for younger, heavier, more active patients because of the improved wear characteristics. Ceramics are most commonly used on the ball-side of the joint but can be used in conjunction with a cup made of plastic, metal, or other ceramics.

The final class of materials used in hip bearing surfaces which I'll discuss here are metals. For many years, we have used a metal ball, but there has been an increasing trend toward using a metal socket as well—the so called metal-on-metal combination. One benefit is that the wear is so small that it's almost un-measurable. This allows for use in younger, heavier, and more active patients. The down side is that there are relatively high levels of metal ions generated by these two metal surfaces rubbing together over the years. Cobalt and Chromium are heavy metals that are mixed with steel to create the alloy that is used most commonly in hip replacement bearing surfaces. These heavy metals must be excreted through the kidneys and there has been concern that a build-up of heavy metal ions in a patient's body my increase patients' risk for certain cancers. As I write this, this concern about a link to cancer has not been proven to my satisfaction in our medical journals, but the concern is enough that it is being investigated.

Some patients (especially female patients) may experience an unusual "immune reaction" of sorts to the metal ions produced by the metals rubbing over time. This rare reaction tends to cause inflammation and pain, and sometimes causes bone to dissolve slowly as well. This metal ion response is not an issue if there is a metal ball and a plastic cup, because all of the wear occurs on the softer (plastic) layer of the joint, and hardly any ionic metal particles are generated. But when metals are used as both the ball and the socket in the joint, more metallic particles are generated. There is also concern about what effect heavy metal ions may have on pregnancy, so this type of hip replacement is often avoided in women of child-bearing age. The topic of metal-on-metal hip replacements is a science in evolution. The vast majority of patients with metal-on-metal hip replacements do quite well. The issues I mention above are being investigated currently and their resolution will, of course, drive the popularity of this type of hip replacement going forward.

Another by-product of having better bearing surfaces is that we're able to use a larger ball in the hip replacement. In the 1970-1990s most hip replacements used a metal ball that was between 22mm and 28mm in diameter. The reason for this was to reduce the amount of wear on the plastic cups. Studies at the time showed this to be the optimal size to reduce wear. The problem was that the smaller the ball, the higher the risk that the hip can pop out of joint (dislocate). Now that the newer materials are making their way into hip replacement designs, we can take advantage of the fact that they wear less, and put a bigger ball on the hip replacements we perform. This makes them much more stable. Nowadays, it's not unusual for surgeons to place a ball that is upwards of 30-50 mm in diameter.

What about "partial" hip replacements? Yes, there is such a thing. Partial hip replacements may also be called "hemi-arthroplasty." In this operation, rather than replacing the ball and the socket, only the ball is replaced. This operation is used if you need to have a hip replacement but your (own) socket is still in good shape. This is rare with patients afflicted by arthritis, because arthritis generally affects both the ball *and* the socket. But there are some conditions that only affect the ball (femoral head). One such condition is hip fracture. Recall from ***Chapter 2, Nuts and Bolts of the Hip and Knee*** that the femoral head is connected to the rest of the thighbone by a bridge of bone called the femoral neck. Well, it turns out, for a number of reasons, that if you break your hip along the femoral neck, it is very unlikely to heal successfully. In this population of patients, it has been shown to be a much better solution to replace just the ball and femoral neck with a partial hip replacement. Assuming the patient did not have hip arthritis before the hip was broken, the cup should be in fine shape and therefore not in need of replacement. Or put another way, "If it ain't broke don't fix it."

There is another type of hip replacement called *hip resurfacing.* Hip resurfacing is used mainly for younger and more active patients for reasons that we will discuss here. The idea behind hip resurfacing is that only the *natural surfaces* of the joint need to be replaced because this is presumably the source of the pain in diseased hips. The parts of a hip resurfacing implant, rather than being an entire ball and socket, can be thought of as thin "caps" which are placed on the existing ball and socket. In this operation, rather than remove and replace the femoral head and neck, the bones are shaped appropriately by the surgeon, and a cap is placed over the existing bone. This allows for a larger head to be used (remember the larger the head is, the less likely the hip is to dislocate). It also allows for the patient to keep more of his own bone (because we are simply capping, rather than replacing, the femoral head and neck). This could theoretically make any future surgery easier and more successful for your surgeon, because he would have more of your own natural bone to work with. With this type of hip replacement, a larger femoral head can be placed and therefore the risk of dislocation is low. There is also virtually no issue with leg length differences after this type of surgery.

Every different procedure has its own set of pros and cons. The down sides of hip resurfacing are that they are typically not performed as a minimally-invasive procedure.

158

In fact, the incisions and tissue dissection for hip resurfacings are generally bigger than those required for standard hip replacement. The surgery usually takes longer to perform, and is more technically demanding for the surgeon than a standard total hip replacement. There have also been a few patients undergoing this operation who have broken the hip through the femoral neck after surgery (remember, in this operation the patient keeps their own femoral neck, whereas in a standard hip replacement the femoral neck is replaced with a metal one). Standard hip replacements are also of such high quality these days, that it's unclear whether performing this bigger, more technically demanding operation—with a slightly higher complication rate—is worth the theoretical benefit. Again, this is a science in evolution, so the answers to these questions will become more and more apparent over time.

Knee Replacement Variations

Knee replacement designs, like hip replacement designs, have been driven to evolve based on durability. Obviously, we all want knee replacements to last *longer*. For that reason, in ways similar to those described concerning the hip, we look at materials that are harder and smoother. The knee implants themselves are generally made of either steel alloys or titanium, which are then polished to a high sheen. The spacer is almost exclusively made of *ultra-high molecular weight polyethylene* (UHMW) plastic, or "poly" for short. The poly spacer between the components is the bearing component, and because it is softer than the metal, this is the part that usually wears out first. Research into the durability of implants therefore focuses on two things: how to make the plastic tougher and more wear-resistant, and how to make the metal components smoother so they don't wear out the plastic.

The plastics used in knee replacements today are much more wear-resistant than the plastics used even a decade ago. Advances in the manufacturing have made the poly more durable and wear-resistant without making them so hard and brittle that they are prone to crack. The advances have been mostly in the manufacturing process and were discussed above in the context of hip replacement design materials. The loading pattern and forces in a knee are a bit more complex than that of the hip and so the materials have to be able to withstand these stresses better. The techniques of cross-linking and reduction of oxidation through the use of manufacturing processes has helped reduce wear tremendously.

The smoothness of the metallic components has improved over time as well. One approach has been to coat the surface of the metal implants with a hardened ceramic.

Ceramics can be smoother than metals because of their material properties. The idea is that the less abrasive the components are, the less likely that they are to wear out the plastic inserts. As a result of these complex loading conditions, and the fact that ceramics are generally more brittle, the knee replacement implants employing ceramics are *coated* with the ceramic rather than being solid ceramic throughout.

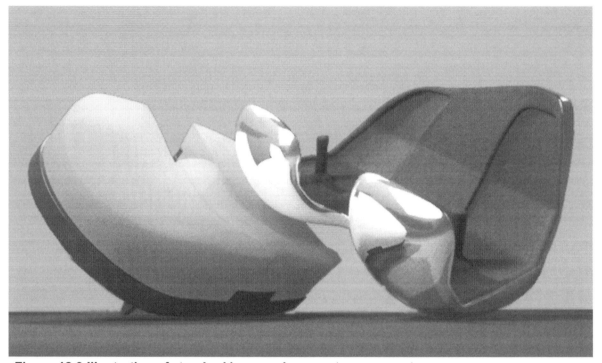

Figure 12.3 Illustration of standard knee replacement components

As we will discuss in ***Chapter 15, What Can Go Wrong?***, *loosening* can occur with knee replacements. This is important because loose components can cause pain and sometimes require revision surgery to correct. Loosening occurs when the parts of the knee replacement are no longer solidly affixed to the bone. In general, there are two methods that we use to get the implant to stick to the bone during knee replacement. The first is to use a type of cement called "methylmethacrylate" to help adhere the knee replacement components to the bone. The other method is a "press fit." A press fit is achieved when you shape the end of the bone and then impact the component into place. No cement is used with this technique. If the bone is shaped properly, the component will "lock" onto the end of the bone and your bone will eventually grow onto (or into) the component to make it stable. Both methods are used today but the cement method is still a bit more common.

Over the last few years, however, new materials have been developed that allow bone to grow in them and through them with relative ease. As these materials improve, I predict that we'll be shifting away from the use of the cement and more toward the implants that are press fit into place. As of the writing of this handbook, the materials and methods for implanting press fit components are under evolution and either cementing or press fitting are acceptable options.

We're always trying to improve the stability and range of motion of knee replacements. We want our patients to have a good functional range of motion in their knee, and have a knee that feels solid under them as well. Remember, the knee replacement components are only a small part of that equation, though an obvious and vitally important part. Proper installation, alignment, genetics, scarring, and physical therapy all play major roles in achieving motion and stability after surgery. The implants help with stability and range of motion based on their shapes. There are literally dozens of different types of knee replacements out there, each with a slightly different shape, and *each one* claiming to be the best. In reality, however, the differences are subtle, and most of the major implant manufacturers have excellent knee replacement designs. With the right mix of technical skill on the part of the surgeon, and good old-fashioned hard work in PT after surgery on the part of the patient, most knee replacement designs will give you excellent range of motion and stability.

I want to also mention an alternative knee replacement design that is appropriate in some cases. The "partial knee replacement" is an implant designed to replace only a specific part of your knee joint. Remember that in **Chapter 2, Nuts and Bolts of the Hip and Knee** we discussed briefly the three "compartments," or areas, of the knee: medial, lateral, and patello-femoral. In the vast majority of patients with arthritis, all three of these areas of the knee joint are affected by arthritis. There are some unusual cases when only one of the three compartments of the knee is worn. If such is the case, there are joint replacements made to replace only that area of your knee joint that is worn out. The advantage is that the surgery is less invasive and your recovery is quicker.

Again, this is unusual. I would say for every one hundred patients I see with arthritis, ninety-five of them have arthritis in all areas of their knees and are not candidates for partial knee replacement. If your X-rays and symptoms suggest that only one of the three areas of your knee is worn out, your surgeon will discuss this option with you. Partial knee replacements have been around in mainstream use since the 1970s, so they're not new. Over the years, they've fallen in and out of favor among the orthopedic surgery community for a variety of reasons. Currently if you're one of the unusual folks in which the arthritis is limited to one area of you knee's joint, I do think it is reasonable to at least consider a partial replacement.

As you can see, the evolving world of total joint replacement can be confusing. You should find a good surgeon with whom you communicate well, and use him as a source of

161

information for discussion. This chapter of our handbook is not meant to be exhaustive in description of the variations on implant design and installation. The goal here is to get you into the conversation, let you know what's out there, and help you learn the ropes when it comes to total and partial joint replacement. Use this information as a springboard for discussions with your surgeon about the various implants and techniques used every day, bearing in mind (as we discussed earlier) that newer does not always mean better. It will be at least a decade before we know if the technology and techniques in use today are better than those used ten years ago. The advancements are made logically and should improve outcomes—but this is not a guarantee. My advice to you is the same as the advice I received from one of my mentors during my many years of training (and I quote): "Dr. Hugate, you should never be the first one onto, nor the last one off of, the bandwagon with any of these implants!" This sage advice has served me well.

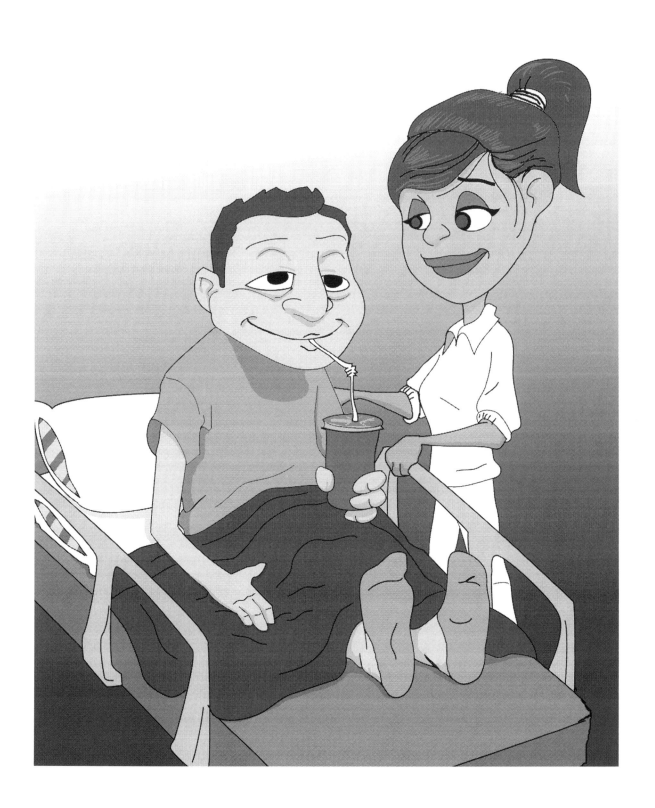

The Hospital Stay

by Robert Holland

In the Recovery Room

I begin this chapter when I'm waking up after surgery. There is an altered awareness in those first few moments that reminds me of the story of Moses where they find a baby floating on the Nile River—only I'm the baby and the Nile River is the recovery room. There's an absolute feeling of helplessness and total dependence on the PACU nurses. Then there's the rediscovery of the people around me as they first discover I'm waking up. It's always hard to remember those first minutes when waking up, but for me, it's always a very fine moment. The first thing I'm aware of are the sounds that surround me. I'm not conscious enough to be thinking words just yet, but sounds come to me as from a distance. There are the beeps and whirrs of medical monitoring devices, the soft murmuring voices of the nurses as they go about their business, and the sounds of other people being brought into and taken out of the recovery room. It's all very dream-like and blurry. Of course, I'm never certain how much time goes by because this is a time for dreamy dozing.

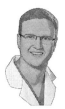

Hugate's Comment: We decided to write this chapter primarily from Robert's point of view. The hospital stay should be a patient-centered experience. For that reason, Robert's thoughts, descriptions, and ideas will take center stage here and I will intersperse comments where I think they will be helpful to you.

Remember, Robert is describing his personal hospital experience in this chapter. While yours will be very similar, it will not be exactly the same. The basic elements of any hospital stay are well represented here. Robert is an excellent writer and if you read his descriptions carefully I'm confident that you'll be mentally prepared for this stage of your recovery. ~*~

After a time, however, it is my awareness of the sounds from the general hustle and bustle of the recovery room that lifts me up into my other senses. There is the antiseptic smell of the hospital bed and plastic tubes attached to me, and the odd aftertaste of unknown pharmaceuticals in my system and the tube they had put in my mouth to help me breathe while Dr. Hugate operated on me. There is cold, fresh air in the recovery room, but my nurses have bundled me with warm blankets and I'm as snug as a bug in a rug. My mouth is dry, so the first thing I ask for (when I finally find my voice) is a sip of water or soda-pop. The recovery room nurses are both very busy and very attentive. I suspect they've been watching me quite closely to see when I'm coming to because, by the time I realize I'd like a drink, they are right there speaking softly to me and welcoming me back. They are my guardian angels, and believe me when I affirm that when I'm lying there flat on my back, all bundled up and looking up into their beautiful, caring eyes—I can see that they are angels indeed. Of course their extensive training (and the various monitoring equipment I'm hooked up to) tells them I'm doing fine, but there is that first *human* moment when I can see the caring in their eyes and know I'm safe.

As I awaken further, I become more and more aware of my surroundings. I now notice the urinary catheter that was inserted during the beginning of the surgery. Apparently, it was placed after I was under anesthesia, because I don't remember it being inserted. It continuously drains my bladder. This is one less thing for me to worry about. There is also something else I notice as I come awake. There are inflatable, elongated tubes (like long blood pressure cuffs) around my calves, surrounding them like cocoons. Attached to them, lying on the foot of my bed, is an air-pump machine about the size of a briefcase and it slowly and gently fills the tubes around my calves with air, squeezing them firmly, and then slowly deflating, all in a continuous cycle. The purpose of this unit, called a *sequential compression device (SCD)*, is to help make the blood in my legs circulate. My knee is wrapped with ACE Wrap (aka ACE Elastic Bandage) and gauze. The nurses have already placed my knee in the continuous passive motion machine (CPM) and it moves my new knee joint back and forth gently.

The next stage of my recovery is marked by two questions which commingle in my mind as I wake up: "How did everything go?" and "Did I need a transfusion?"

The nurse's response: "Everything went fine Robert, and no, you didn't need a transfusion." The recovery room nurse's job is to manage my return to consciousness and make sure that I needn't worry about anything except gathering my senses. She will also tell me what information Dr. Hugate may have given her regarding the surgery. There is a running conversation now where she asks me a question or two, then goes about her business for a bit then comes back and asks me something else. The questions go something like this:

Do you feel nauseated?

Do you want something to eat or drink?

Are you warm enough?

Would you like to have your head elevated a bit?

Again, I'm sure this running conversation has more going on than my comfort.

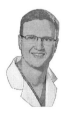

Hugate's Comment: *Robert describes in superb detail his senses as he comes out of anesthesia: the sights, the sounds, and even the smells. His experiences here are typical for a patient recovering from "general anesthesia": a "twilight" or "dream-like" state in which time perception may be lost. The experience will be slightly different for those undergoing different types of anesthesia.*

The recovery room nurses are an experienced and compassionate breed of nurse and here they watch Robert closely for signs of recovery. The nurses receive a report from the surgeon and the anesthesiologist as Robert enters the recovery room about how the surgery went, and how he did medically throughout the procedure. They convey this information to Robert once he's awake enough to perceive and process it.

The main goal of the nurses in the recovery room is to ensure that Robert's "systems" are all coming back on-line—that is, his heart, lungs, and thought-processing systems. The nurses make careful note of the interactions they have with Robert as he awakens, and the level of these interactions determines when Robert is ready to move out of the recovery room. Of course, he is closely monitored and his operative leg is checked frequently. As you will now see, warmth, pain, and nausea tend to be the "comfort issues" dealt with most frequently in the recovery room. Communication with your nurse is crucial, as they have lots of tricks for making you comfortable if the need arises. ~*~

An indeterminate period goes by where I'm climbing upwards into wakefulness notwithstanding all the medication still in me. Oddly enough, I'm always a bit hungry—not all that surprising since I've had nothing to eat for more than sixteen hours. So when she asks me if I want some crackers, I say, "Yeah...." For some reason, there is nothing quite as good as a bite and some soda-pop after regaining consciousness post-surgery. Maybe it's an affirmation that goes something like, "I eat, therefore I live!"

During my last TKR, they didn't have my room ready as soon as they wanted, so rather than make my wife stay out in the waiting room, they let her come in to sit beside me. This is another one of those first eye contact moments. I am quite sure that there is no more loving sight than looking up into the eyes of my wife and watching her face flood with relief. To see the tension leave her body as she reaches out to hold my hand and bends over me to give me a big kiss is an affirmation of a successful beginning to our journey. I say "our journey" here because there can be no doubt that my wife, who's my at-home caregiver and biggest stakeholder, is along with me on this float trip with me all the way. Of course, she fusses over me, holds my hand, and doesn't know exactly what to do, but just having her near to me is a kind of miracle—so it's OK, everything is OK....

The next scene in this journey is when my recovery room nurse decides I'm ready to be released to the floor. After I'm done waking up and have been checked and rechecked a few times, my recovery room nurse gives the OK. However, before I can go to my hospital room she calls the floor nurse and checks to see if my room is available and gives a technical report about me to my floor nurse before handing me off. This always serves to reassure me that my floor nurse knows I'm fresh out of surgery, knows how I've been doing, and that this new guardian angel will be watching me closely.

At this point, my recovery room nurse has gone ahead and called those folks who move me about the hospital, who are known as "transport staff." Of course, as we head out of the recovery room, I wave goodbye to my recovery room nurse, and the caravan through the halls begins with me flat on my back in my fancy hospital bed. I am accompanied by all of my machines, monitors, bags of IV fluids, and tubes dangling about from a pole on the side of my bed. With my wife following along watching over me too, it's quite a caravan. This is another one of those surrealistic rides I spoke about in **Chapter 10, The Day of Surgery**, once again traversing the labyrinthine halls of the hospital from the recovery room to my hospital room while flat on my back. Finally, we arrive at my room where next I get to meet my floor nurse. At this point, my care officially transfers from the recovery room nurse to the floor nurse, who'll be taking care of me post-surgery for the next few hours.

As you read on in this chapter, you will notice that I spend an inordinate amount of time describing the first night after surgery and the following day. This is because I'm generally writing about things in order that they occurred. As I write, I will also stop periodically and explain about meeting my caregivers, explain what they do, and cover the equipment and various devices that are part of my recovery. This will help you get a sense of the overall picture of your own recovery while in the hospital. What I'm not doing is trying to supplant this handbook for the many years of education and expertise each one of my caregivers went through to be where I need them. As such, I will attempt to describe their functions as I perceive them while Dr. Hugate fills in any gaps.

The most unfamiliar period of time to me in my journey through the hospital was the first twenty-four hours. After that, everything settles into a kind of routine whose purpose is to get me up, get me moving, and prepare me for discharge. As such, I'll relate my story about the events, people, and experiences almost as if it's a journal, chronicling my journey through total joint replacement.

The Rest of the Day

Before I know it, I'm wheeled into my room where the floor nurse assumes responsibility, and yes, this is another of those eye-contact moments. As I first look into her eyes, I'm always amazed at the kindness and compassion there—it's a very nice (if not a bit hectic) moment—there's lots going on. The first thing I notice about the new bed they want me in, is a strong metal bar overhead (from head to foot) which has a height-adjustable, triangular trapeze hanging down **(See Figure 13.1)**. They have me grab hold of this trapeze and use it to help

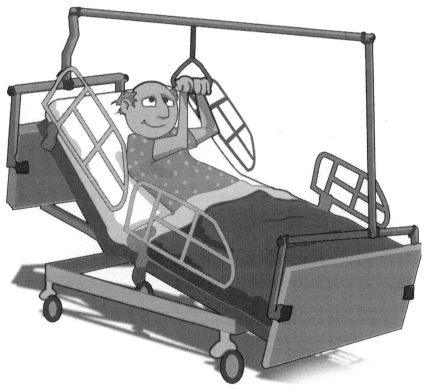

Figure 13.1 Cartoon "Man alive! This trapeze-thingy sure is nice for moving around when my backside gets sore! Can't wait until I get back up walking again!"

them move me across and onto my new bed. I'll be using this handy gadget a lot throughout the next few days. Without calling for help, I can pull myself up if I slip downward, and shift my body around when my back gets sore. Also, all of the various hospital staff have me use it whenever they need me to lift myself up (or move about) for whatever reason. It's truly wonderful, but requires a bit of upper body strength and I'm glad I work out at the gym about once a week.

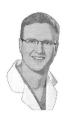

Hugate's Comment: *Robert again brings up a good point here that I would like to elaborate on. The better your strength is going into surgery, the easier your recovery will be. Here, he discusses specifically the ability to move about in bed immediately after surgery using the overhead trapeze. This is highly dependent on both upper body strength and the strength of your other (non-operative) leg. Your ability to transfer will be greatly improved if you have strengthened your arms, shoulders, and legs prior to surgery—but this is not the only benefit of good strength. You will also improve your abilities to get up and walk safely with the physical therapist, reduce your risk for falls, and require less effort on the part of people helping you at home after surgery. For these reasons, I recommend that anyone considering hip or knee replacement surgery discuss this with your primary care provider. If you are healthy enough, and your PCP agrees, then consider a light strengthening routine far enough in advance of surgery to be of help. ~*~*

As I start to settle in, I begin to notice a few more items in my room. There is a monitor pole next to my bed. It's about six feet tall and mounted on wheels. It's kept in the room with me, and an array of small monitoring devices, IV pumps, and other medical equipment are mounted on it, making it resemble a high-tech totem pole. One monitor in particular is a machine about the size of a toaster. This complex machine is attached to the blood pressure cuff on my arm and has a screen and lots of buttons and dials. It's responsible for collecting my vital signs (blood pressure and pulse), which it does by automatically inflating the cuff on my arm every so often. It will make a loud (and somewhat startling) beeping noise if my blood pressure is not within the appropriate range. This can be heard by the staff and they'll come a-running right away to find out what's the matter. The machine also has a little gizmo that resembles a clothes-pin that clamps gently onto one of my fingers and is attached to the same monitor by a small wire. Its job is to constantly sense my *oxygen saturation levels* to make sure I'm breathing as well as I ought to be.

This brings us to *the machine*! "Yikes!" you say, "What is *the machine*?" It's known as a continuous passive motion machine or CPM. The CPM is a device that lies underneath my entire lower limb (operative side), cradles it lengthwise, and cycles up and down under the new knee (**See Figure 13.2**). This complex, mechanical unit slowly flexes and extends my knee to keep it from stiffening. The CPM was first placed on my knee in the recovery room immediately after surgery. It will be taken off overnight, to allow me to rest, and is then reapplied in the morning about an hour after breakfast. Dr. Hugate has ordered that I use the CPM at least six hours a day. Now that the surgery is over, regaining the range of motion of this new knee is now the foremost consideration. It will be the focus of much intensive effort for the next couple of months. Remember that while bending my new knee soon after surgery is obviously very important, so is straightening it—in fact, straightening my operative leg is even more important! As for me, I always feel it helpful to keep one thought foremost in my mind:

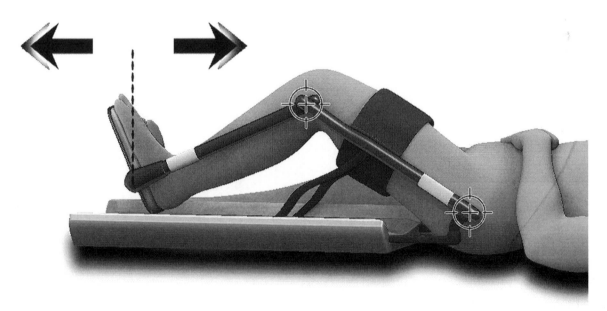

Figure 13.2 Illustration of CPM (continuous passive motion machine)

This whole journey I've undertaken through joint replacement is about motion, mobility, and regaining the freedom of living without constant, debilitating pain in my daily life.

So I make sure I'm in the CPM enough hours during the day to satisfy Dr. Hugate's orders, and so do my floor nurses.

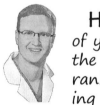

Hugate's Comment: Robert is right on here. Getting through the surgery is only half the battle. Without further efforts at regaining your motion, the surgery will fail. These efforts will involve the CPM machine (if you had knee replacement), the physical therapists, and some home exercises going forward. The whole point of going through this process is to regain your function and reduce your pain. Don't short change yourself by "coasting" after surgery. It will make the process all for naught. Prepare yourself mentally for hard work before you go into surgery. After surgery, find the strength to keep charging forward. ~*~

At this point, my floor nurse begins to assess me and also delivers a briefing to instruct me about *the plan* for the next few days. Dr. Hugate has left orders for (among other things) pain medications, and my floor nurse goes over this with me now. She begins our dialogue with queries like, "Are you in pain? Do you want supper? How do you feel?" While asking all of these important questions, she's taking my vital signs as well. She checks my body temperature, blood pressure, oxygen saturation, eye response, IV connections, pulse, my bandages, and such—all to get an overall picture of how I'm doing and—you guessed it—hooking me up to my monitor pole.

Hugate's Comment: One thing the nurses measure as part of your vital signs is your level of pain. Pain is subjective, and so the scoring of pain accounts for that. The nurse will ask you to rank your pain on a scale of one to ten. Be honest. There is nothing glorious about being in pain. Every once in a while I get patients who try to "tough out" the pain, and they do themselves a tremendous disservice. If you understate your pain level to the nurse, you may not receive adequate pain medications. And once you fall behind on your pain control, it will be difficult to catch back up. So don't try to be stoic. It is not a sign of strength to refuse pain medications after surgery—it's a sign of foolishness. Rest assured, the pain medications are ordered in such a way that will not cause overdose and will not result in you becoming addicted (which are common concerns on the part of my patients). Please take advantage of the many options your doctor has ordered for pain management. ~*~

As another part of the plan, my nurse describes to me the various methods and devices used to track my fluid status after surgery—the "ins-and-outs" tracking. The concept is simple: if the medical team knows how much fluid is *leaving* my body, and how much fluid is *entering* my body, they can make sure that I do not become either dehydrated or over-hydrated. Recall the urinary catheter? It is an important part of the ins-and-outs equation. It is connected by a small tube to a bag hanging from the side of the bed that collects urine. This bag has graduated marks on it, such that, until the urinary catheter comes out, my caregivers can see exactly how much water my body is processing.

The other basic tools of the ins-and-outs arsenal are introduced to me as follows: a one-liter plastic pitcher, a plastic-cup, and a urinal bottle with closeable top that will be useful after the catheter is removed. Each of these items has markings to allow the nurses to measure how much fluid is in the vessel. (Incidentally, these items are mine to keep as part of the nifty "goodie bag" I get for entering the hospital) The nurses and the nurse's aides are all very diligent about this tracking. They write down how much fluid gets put into the graduated pitcher, how much goes into me through my IV, and so on. If they bring me a can of soda-pop or a carton of cranberry juice, they track that too. Note that no one other than the nurse or the nurse's aide is to fill the little pitcher or empty the urinal so my fluid intake and output can be tracked accurately.

This raises another issue: bowel movements (or BMs). BMs are also an integral part of the ins-and-outs equation and therefore must be recorded. If you feel the need to have a bowel movement, let your nurses know before it becomes urgent. Even if it's a false alarm, be proactive and call for assistance anyway. Here's why: the action of trying to create a BM signals your body to keep the processes in operation. With all the pharmaceuticals and time in bed, on your back, your body needs these signals to get back in the game. Remember that constipation adds a whole layer of complexity to what is already a rather difficult time.

Next, my floor nurse explains that we must be very diligent about keeping the operative site cool ("operative site" is the term used by your doctor to indicate the knee or hip that was operated on). The operative site tends to get warm due to inflammation from the surgery and usually swells up. Keeping the site cool is very important in reducing inflammation and swelling after surgery. As soon as I'm settled in, she puts a rather large bag of ice on my knee. This routine is something I find extremely helpful as it also significantly reduces the pain. I can tell you, when the ice is melted and my leg warms up a bit, it starts to hurt and throb. I call my nurse or her aide: "Time for more ice!"

There are other items in the take-home "goodie bag" besides those for ins-and-outs measuring. They are generally the following: a toothbrush and toothpaste; a curved plastic basin; some warm and fuzzy, non-slip sock-booties; a small box of tissues for nose blowing; and a cute little plastic tub. Each of these take-home goodies is there for a purpose. They don't want me bringing my own toothbrush with me as it might bring with it some germs from home. The sock-booties are to keep my feet warm because the nurses will be getting me in and out of bed (much sooner than I think or want them to), and they don't want me to slip or fall. The tub is for washing up. The curved plastic basin is for use in case I get nauseous or need to spit. I was allowed to bring my robe and some house slippers from home, and I use the robe when I'm cleared to go up and down the halls with my walker, so I'm not "mooning" the people behind me! (Those hospital gowns can be very revealing.)

Let's go back and revisit the hospital bed and my hospital room. These days, the hospital bed is a marvel of modern science and technology. It can raise and lower to help the staff care for you without having to bend over all of the time. It can bend up or down in supporting your upper body and flex up under your knees as much as you want. For me, after so many years in heavy construction, my lower back gives me fits when lying flat, so this is darn good. Some elevation of the head of the bed and under my knees can be very comforting, even necessary. These new beds can also have many other controls built-in, such as a nurse call button, and a special bar to hold the IV bag and hoses (although once I begin moving about they switch me to an IV pole like the one in **Figure 13.3**). They also have the overhead bar and trapeze I spoke about earlier, and sometimes even television controls. Depending on the hospital you're in, the beds may be a bit simpler, but they will still have the capability of raising and lowering your upper body and knees on command. One thing all of these beds also have in common is a set of rails on either side which keep you from rolling off the side of the bed and falling on the floor (**See Figure 13.1**). There is usually a stainless steel panel behind the head of the bed which is there for other esoteric purposes; for instance, as a feed for oxygen, a connection for suction devices, and hookups for other specialized equipment.

Hugate's Comment: A piece of equipment that Robert does not mention here is a PCA (Patient Controlled Anesthesia) device. Many surgeons, including me, order these devices to be used for the day after surgery when pain control can be the most difficult. Because of the type of anesthesia Robert received, he did not need a PCA, but they are commonly used. The PCA is a hand-held, push-button that is connected to a pump on the monitor/IV pole assembly (the "high-tech totem pole" Robert mentioned above). When you press this button, a predetermined amount of pain medication is measured and delivered into your system through the IV. The device is programmed so as to only deliver that medication ordered, and not to allow you to overdose yourself. The benefit of a PCA is that you control exactly when and how much pain medication is administered without having to call the nurses for each individual dose. It's very important that only the actual patient control the PCA device. On occasion, a patient's family member or friend will try to help by pushing the button for the patient. This can be very dangerous and even lead to an overdose. One of the inherent, protective mechanisms of a PCA is that the patient must be awake and alert enough to push the button for himself. If a patient is not aware enough to hit his own PCA button, then he shouldn't be receiving additional pain medication. Keep this button in an easy-to-find location for the first twenty-four hours after surgery and use it as frequently as needed to manage your pain—that's why it's there. ~*~

In my room, there is also a white dry-erase board on the wall which identifies me to anyone who comes into my room for any reason. Part of that elaborate system of identity crosschecks Dr. Hugate spoke about earlier, this board helps to make sure I get my own medications (versus somebody else's), to ensure that the lab technician draws blood from the right person, and so on. So the board will display my name, any allergies, and any especially important orders from my physicians. It also displays my caregiver's names (including both doctor's and nurse's name) and anything else that may be especially important to my case. Many hospitals also display here the phone number for the hospital's patient advocate, should I need her services.

Almost all hospitals have televisions mounted in each room. My TV was mounted up on the wall, out of the way, and didn't have the built-in speaker enabled. To listen to the programs of my choice, I've got a TV controller of some sort (either built into my bed or coming from the control panel and built into the hand unit) and it has a little speaker built in with a private volume control. This is so I don't keep my neighbor awake, whether I'm in a private room or not.

It's getting to be about suppertime by now and I've been napping and watching a bit of TV with my wife sitting faithfully beside me. The hospital wait staff brings me my first meal. The meal delivery person (one of my favorite people) leaves a menu for the next day's meal order. The nurses may limit what I'm allowed to eat depending on whether I have any other special conditions (like heart disease, diabetes, and so on) or allergies to be concerned about. Hospitals have gotten some bad raps for having unpalatable food, but these days, I have found that everything is very good and I know there is a nutritionist somewhere who's keeping a watchful eye on my every dietary need. Of course, I keep in mind any self-imposed dietary restrictions from home, but I also know that my stay here is going to be very challenging. I take every opportunity to make it as enjoyable and pleasant as possible. For me, there is a time and a place to diet. I think it wise to remember that I've just undergone a very serious surgery and here is a chance to rejoin life and celebrate my success. So I'll diet later and indulge now—within reason of course—and I keep in mind that eating tasty foods is one of the most basic joys in life.

Hugate's Comment: I agree with Robert. Yes, there is a time and a place to diet, and this isn't it. After surgery, your body becomes highly catabolic (meaning your metabolism increases and you need extra calories to heal from surgery). Of course there will be certain restrictions if you have a history of heart disease, diabetes, or similar conditions. But in the absence of specific dietary restrictions, I allow my patients to eat the foods they enjoy after surgery. Not only does it give them the calories they need during recovery, it also makes them feel more and more like a human being again. ~*~

This brings us near to a close for the first night after surgery and my introduction to a host of strange devices and other odd experiences. As I lay there, all cozy in my hospital room, I am very sleepy. My beautiful wife is sitting next to me so worried and yet so relieved. It's finally the end of a long day, and finally time to relax. When visiting hours are over, I encourage my wife to go on home before it gets too late. During this first night after surgery I notice (even though the nurse thinks I'm asleep) that they check on me frequently, and I have some sense of their comings and goings. Everything is strange: the sights, the sounds, the smells, the bed, the medications, and even the temperature of things around me. This all combines to make the first night a very out-of-the-ordinary experience. Be assured, I feel very safe because I have a call button to alert my nurse. Nowadays there is an intercom built into the call button so that when I push the button, somebody answers (via the intercom) to ask me what I need. This is so the nurse (or the nurse's aide) doesn't have to make a possibly unnecessary trip to the room. If I need something, I call, they answer, and soon everything is taken care of.

Before I move on to describe the next several days after surgery, let's talk about the importance of communications:

You have it within your power to make the experience of communicating with all the hospital's caregivers a positive and pleasant experience.

176

Naturally, when you've had a surgery as serious as a knee or hip joint replacement, you can very easily become cranky, or get to feeling the blues. I have, so I know. If you simply let the staff know how you're feeling, *instead of acting-out on your feelings*, you'll undoubtedly do better and so will they. Remember, the staff is human too. If you are rotten, mean, and nasty, how do you think they'll behave toward you? You have it within your power to bring out their best, or polarize them with bad behavior and watch them turn into the "nurse of steel" (not good). So here's some wisdom about nurses: they must manage you and your care, they're charged with your well-being, and they take their duties very seriously. What else would you expect (or want)? Simply put:

We all have rights and we all deserve to be treated with kindness, dignity, and respect.

If you're hurting, or feeling blue and you snipe or bark at them, take a moment and say, *"I'm sorry, I'm not myself."* Make an effort to be kind and you'll be pleasantly surprised at how another human being responds when she realizes that you're down in the dumps yet still trying to be a courteous and pleasant human being. Having said all this, personality conflicts can occur. If this takes place, and you feel you cannot cope, or feel uncomfortable to a large extent with your caregiver, speak to the patient advocate rather than getting into a feud. You can always be assigned a different nurse—it may be better for you both.

Hugate's Comment: These are important points here so I will comment just to underscore. As with any interpersonal interaction, it all comes down to open and fair communication. It is simply human nature that patients can become cranky after surgery and bark at their caregivers. It is also human nature that nurses will take better care of patients (and pay more attention to patients) whom they find to be friendly and enjoyable to be around.

If there's an issue that you simply cannot resolve with your caregiver, the appropriate next step is to contact the floor's "charge nurse." This nurse is the leader of that shift and can often take care of any issues you have with your care or with any caregivers you may not be getting along with.

If the issue is still not remedied to your satisfaction after discussing it with the charge nurse, the next step is to contact the hospital's patient advocate. This person's job is to listen to your complaints and advocate for you in an effort to resolve them. He is on your side and can often act as a liaison between you and the staff to get issues worked out. It is rare that

177

the patient advocate is necessary to resolve disputes, but he is there if you need him. If the phone number is not plainly displayed in your hospital room, then simply dial the hospital operator and ask to be connected to the patient advocate—this is a valuable resource. ~*~

The First Day (after surgery)

I think I'm entitled to sleep in after being operated on the day before—but as it turns out, I'm not. Long before the sun rises, Robert rises (that'd be me)! In the wee hours, just before the sun starts to chase the darkness of night away and brightens on the horizon— when I'm sleeping like a log—somebody comes into my hospital room and rousts me awake. It starts with a technician taking an EKG (electro-cardiogram). She places some sticky pads to the skin on my chest and hooks the pads, via tiny wires, to their machine to look at my heart function. Next, there's another technician who wants a blood sample to check my blood count and clotting factors (and whatever else Dr. Hugate is monitoring my blood for). Then, a nurse hustles in and takes a urine sample from the catheter bag. Somebody else shows up with a paper cup of pills I'm supposed to take. They all check my whiteboard to make sure I'm me—and I'm pretty sure I am. They also check my hospital bracelet to ensure my identity. Do you get the picture here? It's a very hectic and early morning. After this seemingly rude (yet in fact very benign) awakening, and after they've all done everything they wanted, checked everything they needed to check, and generally gotten me all woken up—off they all go to roust some other poor soul and do the same things to him. As a side note—it has always amazed me how perky and happy these folks are to roust me awake. In fact, this is a very busy time of the morning for the hospital staff as they check everybody, distribute medications, and make sure all their patients are doing fine.

 Hugate's Comment: I love Robert's description of the first morning after surgery. I've been a patient myself on a few occasions and I can verify that his descriptions are right on. Why do we do this to you? Most doctors make rounds on their patients early in the morning, around 7AM or thereabouts. This is because we have a day full of work ahead of us and this is the "calm before the storm." We all have to either go on to the office and see patients there, or go to the operating room and perform operations during the day. This is often the only time of the day when we can sit down, uninterrupted, take a deep breath, and concentrate on you and all the important details of your recovery. It is therefore critical that we have all of the information that we need during that morning visit to make the critical decisions for the day. Labs, X-rays, vital signs, EKGs, ins-and-outs, and pain scores all help us shape the plan for the day—and therefore must be completed before we see our patients. As you can imagine if I have seven patients in the hospital, and they all have two tests that are not complete in the morning when I see them, I will have to come back again later and look up all fourteen results. I can do this, but it certainly increases the risk that I will not get critical information I may need in a timely fashion to make the appropriate plan for the day: it may be 6 p.m. or later before I can get back to the floor and read those results. The take-home message here is: please do not think of the hospital as a hotel. Although we do our very best to make the hospital a pleasant place to be, there will be interruptions to your sleep as we do what we need to take care of you after surgery. As your condition improves, there will be less need for testing and therefore fewer interruptions to your sleep. ~*~

Then my floor nurse comes in and examines me, checking the dressings on my knee, making me wiggle my toes and do ankle exercises (called ankle pumps) by moving my foot and toes up and down. She also pinches and prods my leg here and there to make sure I can feel everything she's touching. She takes all my vitals again, including temperature. I tend to run low-grade fevers after surgery. Then, after everybody is done, they are suddenly gone and there I lay. I have always found it hard to get back to sleep but if I really work at it, I can do so. However, it's good to be awake and watch the first sunrise of the rest of my life. I usually watch the news or something else on the TV, maybe remember to ask for a newspaper, and then, about the time I've started to doze off again, here comes breakfast.

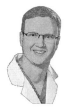 **Hugate's Comment:** Just a brief word here about fevers after surgery. The most common cause for low-grade fever for the first few days after surgery is a condition called "atalectasis." This occurs when your breathing is too shallow, which is quite common after surgery because of immobility and pain medications. The problem here is that parts of the lung can fail to fully expand and this may cause a fever. For this reason, most hospitals issue you an "incentive spirometer." This is a plastic device that has a

179

mouthpiece through which you pull air in order to move a small indicator in the device. This should be used at least ten times per hour while you're awake, completely filling your lungs each time you use it. If you're watching television, use it two to three times each time a commercial comes on and you will meet your quota. If you fill your lungs with air using this device frequently, you will usually find that your temperature comes down to normal within hours.

Of course fever can also be a sign of infection, though infections do not usually cause fevers until five or six days after surgery. Despite this, once the dressing has been removed, we check the wound daily for any signs of infection. Another thing we do routinely is order antibiotics surgery to prevent infection. Most surgeons give a dose of antibiotics just before the operation itself, followed by twenty-four hours of IV antibiotics after the surgery as well. So the likelihood that Robert's fever here (only a day after his surgery) is related to wound infection is very small. ~*~

Sometime about mid-morning, my floor nurse will come in again and check the urinary catheter. If I'm doing well and processing enough of the fluids I'm taking in, she'll remove it. This is more embarrassing than anything else. There is a little pain associated with it, but it is such a relief to gain another step toward freedom of motion once it's out. It's one less tube and one less thing to carry around. Now it's time to start using that plastic urinal. Be proactive about keeping the urinal from getting too full. When it's about two-thirds of the way full, call for it to be emptied. Keep in mind my caregivers are still tracking my ins-and-outs for at least one to two days more, depending on how I'm doing. So until my floor nurse tells me it's OK, even if I can get to the room's toilet myself (usually by the second day), I still have to use the urinal. At this point, it's time to get cleaned up, and I learn how to get a bath in bed. My little plastic washtub is filled with nice hot water and the nurses help me wash up. It's simply exquisite to be getting clean. They help me carefully move about, but here again, the trapeze bar becomes the tool of the day as I shift myself about, helping to expose the backside parts that need scrubbing too.

By now it's mid-morning, and you wouldn't think they'd be in bothering me before lunch—especially to get up out of my nice bed—but you'd be wrong. As the day after surgery begins to really take shape, the physical therapist comes into my room and explains that it is not time to rest. He's carrying a rather complicated, full-length knee brace. This fancy brace bends at the knee and fastens both down by my ankle and well above mid-thigh. It has reinforced sides and a number of possible adjustments and hook-and-loop straps. It is complete with new pads, all designed to wrap around and guide my leg in the correct way needed to protect my new knee. Dr. Hugate has ordered that my leg be in this knee brace when I'm not in the CPM. My physical therapist explains why I have been given this brace: mainly to protect my new joint replacement. Before I know it, he's strapping this brace to my leg and preparing me to get out of my nice, fancy hospital bed—and here I was thinking, "Uh-huh, I'll just be taking it e-e-easy." But no-o-o-o, wrong again!

Hugate's Comment: The use of knee braces after knee replacement surgery is a surgeon's preference. I typically do not order knee braces for my routine knee replacement patients but because Robert's knee replacement was a revision surgery, I ordered him a hinged knee brace. These are mainly used to protect the knee while you are walking and improve your stability. The hinge in Roberts knee brace also offers the ability to bend the knee in the brace while still protecting him. ~*~

As he lifts the blanket back from my leg I notice I've got lots of things attached. Odd that I didn't notice all these little doohickeys before, but the period between the surgery and this seminal moment the following day is already a bit fuzzy. There is a little machine taped to my leg that delivers medication for my nerve block. It's attached to a little tiny tube that's running into my upper thigh under some tape. There is also a knee drain running out from under my new knee's bandages, and the little tube goes into another gizmo taped to my leg that pulls pinkish fluid out from the inside of my new knee. The medical team monitors the amount of fluid being pulled out of the knee joint as an indicator for how much blood loss I may have ongoing after surgery. My PT has to work around all of these tubes as he straps my leg into the knee brace, and soon I'm ready to move. This is when I begin to truly realize that using my newly replaced knee joint is not something I get to wait for.

Physical therapy instructions begin shortly after getting the knee strapped into the brace, and include how to use the trapeze bar to pull myself into a sitting position. Next, the PT lowers the rail on the side of the bed and helps me pivot to where my new knee is sort of sticking straight out in the splint, toes wriggling. Then he puts those warm and fuzzy, non-slip sock-booties on my feet and I realize he's completely serious about standing up. I'm thinking, "Man, this is great," and I say to him, "You don't mean to tell me you want me to walk on this knee do you?" And his answer is, "Why, yes... that's why I'm here, Robert," and he smiles.

Then, he introduces me to the walker. That clever fellow, he spirited a walker in when I wasn't looking and is determined to teach me how to use it right then and there. The walker is a light-weight, folding, four-legged stand (with little wheels on the front legs), designed to allow me to put my weight on it and use it like "mobile handrails" in keeping my balance while learning to walk again. Getting up, sitting down, and walking become the subjects of the next half-hour in which I'm standing there holding on to the darn thing. Of course, he's right beside me, holding me steady as I slowly and gingerly bring my weight to bear on my new leg—helping me, encouraging me, and keeping me safe. This moment begins the first of many serious adventures with my physical therapists.

After what I've been through, I am amazed and surprised at how quickly my caregivers all want me out of bed and moving, but there are many compelling reasons. My body wants to settle, and they don't want that. Everybody wants my body to rise and shine—and I do too, of course. Remember what I said about fiber and all that? The actions of standing up, walking, and sitting down make the food and fiber go through the pipeline. Standing and moving also helps fill my chest with air and gets me off of the pressure points on my backside (which keeps bedsores from forming). My PT also explained to me that he wants me up and moving very soon to reestablish my balance. Wow! All that from just standing up?

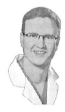 **Hugate's Comment:** I know what you're thinking: "Why are you picking on Robert by making him get up so soon after surgery?" There is a saying in orthopedics that goes way back:

Life is motion! Motion is life!

This statement is true on many levels. Early movement after surgery has been shown to benefit patients in a number of ways. As Robert mentions, constipation can be a big problem after surgery, mostly because of the pain medications and anesthesia medications we give, combined with a lack of mobility. Getting up and moving around is the surest way to get your gut working again and avoid painful constipation.

More importantly, early motion has been shown to help reduce the risk for serious medical conditions such as blood clots, bed-sores, and pneumonia. For these reasons, our goal is to get you up and moving about after surgery as soon and as safely as possible. ~*~

After a bit of time standing with my PT beside me, I'm very happy to lie down again, and he helps me back into my bed. Again, the trapeze bar is excellent for pulling myself back up into bed and positioning myself comfortably. Then, as I settle in and catch my breath after that adventure, here comes lunch. After I eat, things begin settling down and I try to remember what I've learned from my Labrador retrievers: "Always leave time in your schedule for a good nap." In fact, by the time this first morning has passed, I'm completely tired out. My floor nurse wants to get my leg back in the CPM and ice my knee for a couple of hours, and "Oh, yeah—ice is nice."

Campone's Comment: Before hip replacement, there was a part of me that thought I'd never again walk like I did when I was younger when everything worked just fine. My surgery was scheduled early in the day and, like Robert, I had a visit from the PT on that same day in the late afternoon(though I was still very much under the influence of the pain medications and anesthesia, I had been advised in the pre-operative training class that this would be the case). The PT was cheerful, caring, and determined to get me out of bed and over to the chair in my room. She had one of those sneaked-in walkers Robert mentioned, and she showed me, move by move, how I'd be getting out of bed for the next few months. Using the mechanical advantage of the bed, I elevated my head and upper body. The PT then helped me shift into position, carefully inch toward the walker and stand. Amazing— the hip worked! No, I didn't suddenly feel like I was twenty again. However, the experience of motion—however heavily assisted—confirmed for me that the total hip replacement surgery had worked and that I was now on the road to recovering the very positive experience of myself moving in my body like I was once able to do. ~*~

After lunch, a physician comes into my room. I don't know her but she introduces herself and explains that Dr. Hugate has requested that she look in on me. This lady is one of the folks Dr. Hugate calls a *hospitalist*. She goes over my vital signs, checks my chart, and visits with me for about fifteen to twenty minutes and then goes about her business. It was an unexpected visit and I will eventually see her a couple of more times while I'm here. We talked about diet, my health, what vitamins I take, how often I go to the gym, and lots of other seemingly odd subjects. I even remembered to ask her about herself and what her role was on my medical team.

It's very reassuring that not only is Dr. Hugate watching out for me, but he has his friends and colleagues from other specialties keeping a close watch as well.

Hugate's Comment: *This physician was indeed the hospital- ist who visited Robert. I explain the role of the hospitalist in Chapter 7, Your Medical Team. Briefly, she is a medical expert charged with watching Robert's medical health during his stay. If there are issues with blood pressure, fluid balance, blood sugar, and so on, the hospitalists will generally address those. In addition, the hospitalists are in the hospital twenty-four hours a day and seven days a week in most facilities and are therefore immediately available if the nurses have a ques- tion or if there's an emergency. ~*~*

Now it's time to settle down and rest, and rest feels delicious. An incredible amount of my body's energies have been diverted into healing my leg and it feels great to get some pain meds, lay back, feel the wonderful coolness of the ice pack, and let the CPM lull me to sleep. Time passes as I rest, then sometime in late afternoon, here comes that pesky PT again... and he's still smiling. I'm thinking, "Wait, I thought we were done for the day." But no, there's more. So here we go again. He gets me out of the CPM, wraps my leg up in the fancy knee brace, and we do it all again. And, you guessed it, as soon as we get settled back into the bed and get the ice packs back in place, here comes supper. Remember, whenever it's time to get your next day's menu filled out, be sure to manage this task very diligently.

This seems like a good time to talk about company and visitors—you know, the relatives and friends who come to wish you well in your recovery. This first day after surgery is not a good time for the horde to be dropping in. For one thing, I'm still zonked by the pain meds and, as a result, I'm not all that good of a conversationalist. So if they do stop by, they tend to get to visiting amongst themselves while I'm kind of off in dreamy-land trying to rest. Now this is just me, but I have come to a place in these matters where I'm not afraid to ask, "Hey guys, I'm really tired here, maybe you can come back when I'm not so tired out?" A little time with the extended tribe is fine, but when too much time passes, I find I'm weary and need to rest. I rest a lot that first day. This carries me into the evening and it's time to settle, have my leg in the CPM with ice again, and watch the TV with my wife sitting next to me.

The Second Day

Now we are into the rinse-and-repeat cycle of the hospital stay, so instead of reiterating what I've already written about all the machinery and people from the first day for this second day, I'll pick up the differences. My floor nurse has already removed my urinary catheter and if my ins-and-outs are showing that I'm processing fluids normally, the floor nurse will stop tracking them today. What's more is that after the technical staff has completed their morning's work, and I've finished breakfast, I notice that I'm much more alert. I'm wide awake and feeling a lot better than I did yesterday. I still have my femoral nerve block control unit in place, so pain is still very low. After my floor nurse has checked me out and the nurse's aide has helped me bathe, my nurse comes back in and takes off my bandage to see how the whole thing is looking. My first reaction to seeing my leg without all the dressings is surprise. The incision starts just below my knee, continues up across the front, and stops about where my thigh begins.

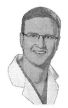

Hugate's Comment: Length of incision is a hot topic in orthopedic surgery for hip and knee replacements. I would say that a six inch incision for knee replacement is about average these days. It used to be that knee replacement incisions were much longer, but with advances in techniques and instruments used during surgery, we can get the length of the incisions down significantly. The length of your incision depends also on the size of your knee: the incision will be slightly larger in bigger patients and slightly smaller in smaller patients. ~*~

So at this point, my nurse cleans the area around my incision and places a new, clean dressing on the leg. I am amazed at the miracle which has just taken place. The worn out and agonizing surfaces of the old knee joint are gone and in their place are some nice, shiny new ones—all mine.

On this second hospital day, the PT comes back in, all smiles as usual, and this time he's ready to do some extended work and training. He removes the bag of ice, helps me out of the CPM, and straps me tightly into the knee brace again. He helps me sit up and pivot, then helps me put my slippers on, and stand up in the walker. Now the instructions shift focus from simply standing and walking a few steps to walking a slightly longer distance. We then go on to learning how to maneuver the walker properly during turns. My first

185

objective is to get to a big easy chair across the room. As to the chair, there it looms in front of me, and it's quite odd what a challenge it seems just to get across that small room, even with a sure and steady PT holding on to me. As I eventually get to the chair and try to sit, he admonishes me not to drop, but rather to put my hands on the armrests and let myself down slowly. Finally, sitting in a chair again! This is a big moment: it's another sign that my life is coming back.

So now I might get to rest, right? No way! Right away my PT wants me to try to lift my leg a few times, wiggle my toes, and gently bend my knee. We then do a few ankle pumps. After about twenty minutes of sitting exercises, I've gotten very tired. Now he asks me if I want to sit a while, and I must admit that sitting for a bit is nice. He promises to come back right after lunch and help me lay down again. Then lunch arrives and I get to eat sitting up in my big hospital easy-chair. It's quite nice to eat sitting up; I'm beginning to feel like myself again. The truth is that on the first day you might not feel much like eating, but on this second day, you will notice some definite need for gustatory delight and will be very glad to have ordered all the things you wanted last night at supper.

After lunch, here comes my new buddy, the physical therapist, just like he promised, and we do some more leg exercises. He now helps me learn how to stand up from a chair with my walker. Now we work our way carefully back over to the bed and he helps me in, and I have to tell you, it feels exquisite to lie back down. We put my leg back in the CPM, call for a bag of ice, and kick back for another afternoon siesta.

This brings us to late afternoon, when I meet my occupational therapist (OT). Occupational therapists specialize in teaching me strategies to perform my routine, everyday activities while recovering from joint replacement. When the OT comes to see me and introduces herself, I already have a good idea of what she is going to cover. Remember the class about total joint replacement that I went to several weeks before the surgery? She was there as an instructor. Now we greet like old friends and she begins asking me about my house: "Do you have stairs? Do you have a shower on the first floor? Are there little doggies, big doggies, kitty cats? Are there little children? Are there other family members besides your spouse?" and so on. (We cover getting your house ready in **Chapter 8, Preparing Your Home**.) She listens, takes notes, and then gives me some materials to read. In truth, she is evaluating me like many of the other caregivers. What seem like friendly questions really have a dual purpose—they also serve to show the staff how my mind is functioning, how my progress is coming, and what they need to do to help me safely return home.

Now the afternoon creeps into evening and I know that soon my wife will be coming to see me and supper will arrive shortly. So we sit there and talk a while and the evening wears away with me out of my CPM and just a nice bag of ice on my knee. Things are definitely getting better.

The Third Day

We have reached the morning of the third day. As each day after surgery goes by, the routine settles in more firmly. Right before sunrise, here comes the technical staff, and by now I know their names, so we visit as they take samples and they do their various tests and whatnot. Then after breakfast, Dr. Hugate comes in and takes the nerve bock out of my thigh, takes my dressings off, and pulls the drain tube out of my knee. Getting all the tubes pulled out always makes me really queasy. I suspect I became a bit pale because Dr. Hugate kids me about it and makes me laugh.

It seems to me that the conversation goes something like this, Dr. Hugate says, "Robert, you've worked hard and are doing well. Your nurses tell me you're a very nice fellow to take care of and they think you have a great sense of humor too. Your PT says you're very determined and the occupational therapist still needs to come in this afternoon and give you her recommendations based on the conversation she had with you yesterday. But, your surgery was a tough one. We had a lot of issues to fix and I don't think you're quite ready to go home yet. What do you think?"

I'm thinking (a task that has become much easier each day as the drugs wear off), "Am I ready to go home? Can I cope with the small stairs in the kitchen? Can I get into the little shower downstairs?" With all this going through my mind, I reply, "Well, you're the Doc, but I think you're right. It seems I get tired really easily and I'm not sure I can pull my weight at home yet."

Dr. Hugate nods his head in a very specific way when he's thinking, and I can almost see the gears turning around in there. "Yes, I think you're right. Let's give you one more night and we'll look at everything again tomorrow—but I think you'll do better at home and right now everything I see tells me you'll be fine. So I'll see you tomorrow morning, and we'll decide." As he walks out of my room I am a bit nervous about the idea of going out from under the wings of all my caregivers.

Hugate's Comment: This is a conversation I have with all of my patients before discharging them. It's important to me that my patients have an idea of when they may go home. This helps them mentally prepare and allows them to activate their going home plan and align their post-surgery caregivers. ~*~

187

Now my friend the PT comes in and he's obviously talked to Dr. Hugate and tells me, "Well Robert, Dr. Hugate tells me I've got to get you ready to go home tomorrow, so let's get to work." Now the physical therapy is much more intense. My PT stands close by but he does not lift my leg out of the CPM for me, nor does he strap my leg into the splint. Rather, he makes me do all of this for myself and watches how I do it and corrects me on this and that. He has me move about the room, over to the sink, and he shows me how to position the walker for hand washing. We then go to the toilet, and he shows me how to employ the walker (to keep me safe when doing my business there). He tells me not to bend down and pick things up, but to use a grabber.

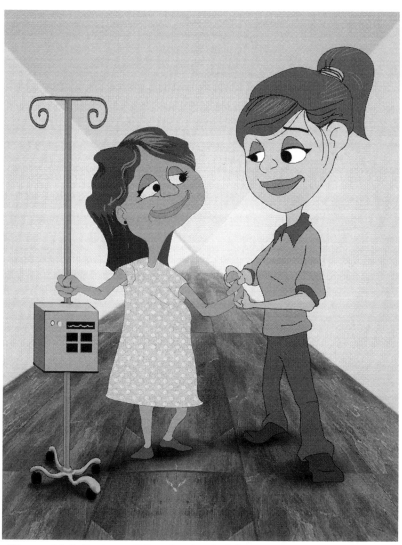

Figure 13.3 Cartoon "Thanks for helping me get up and go for a walk, miss. It's so good to stand up and start moving around again."

Our next adventure is out into the hallway for my first long trek, "Ok, here we go!" So, I'm in my blue terry robe after a nice shave and my hair is brushed, I'm working my way slowly down the hall to the nurse's station, herding my monitor pole along with my PT walking beside me. I have to say, this is one of the finest moments I've ever had. Here I am, walking (albeit with a little help) and my floor nurse looks up from her desk and is totally surprised. You know, I think a little kid resides in all of us down deep inside. My nurse gets up and makes a fuss about how well I'm doing and pats me on the back and I love it—sheesh! It's all very much like when I was in second grade and had just managed to draw a fire engine. Now with the accolades over, everybody goes swiftly back to work. We make our way back down the hall, and as we go my PT tells me not to overdo it, but he tells me that if I want to, I can get myself up and trundle up and down the hall as long as somebody is beside me.

Tired out after all this, I take a nice nap. Then, my OT visits and she has medical equipment and a folder with diagrams based on our interview yesterday. She shows me how to put my socks on with a foot-sized tube called a "sock-puller" (**See Figures 13.4 and 13.5**), which has straps about 3 feet long. I stretch my sock over it, then (using the long straps) I stick my foot in and pull—nice as you please—my sock slides on far enough up my foot and past my ankle that I can reach it and pull it on up. She has a grabber and some crutches and proceeds to teach me how to use them both too. We even go out to the stairwell, and she instructs me how to use either crutches (and/or walker) when ascending and descending stairs. She teaches me how to sit on the edge of my bed to put my underwear and trousers on, and so it goes. The practical applications last about 2-3 hours, during which, some of them I get to try, and others I'm not quite ready for. She promises to return tomorrow and we'll practice the stairs again before I get to go home and she also admonishes me to practice a bit (carefully) on my own because she can't release me for discharge before I master my ADL requirements. The rest of the afternoon is spent between sitting in my CPM while icing my knee, and practicing getting my new splint on. While waiting for my wife to arrive (so she can walk me up and down the hall), I also practice getting in and out of bed and going over to the big chair. Then my hospitalist comes to go over my progress. Whew—that's a lot for one day!

Optional Fourth Day

This big day starts like every other day here, with the hospital technicians waking me up at the crack of dawn. Today my floor nurse comes in and runs through her daily checklist. She then disconnects me from the monitor pole, changes my dressings, and looks everything over. It's all very much like friends saying goodbye. She even gives me a hug. It is at this moment that I realize I have created a bond with all of my caregivers. I guess it makes sense, they've just guided—and assisted—me through one of the most serious adventures I've ever been on in my life, and I never left the building. Therefore, I will use this moment to say:

Thanks to all the people who helped me after my surgery.

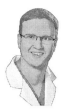

Hugate's Comment: The length of time in the hospital depends on a number of factors: age, health, functional abilities, home conditions, how much help is available at home, the complexity of the surgery, and so on. We do not want to send anyone home who is not prepared to go. Our basic criteria for discharging patients is that they are functioning independently with ADLs (activities of daily living), their pain is under control with oral pain medications, they are able to tolerate food, and they are able to urinate on their own without a catheter. Some of these determinations are subjective and some objective. When I decide to send someone home, it's only after conferring with the therapists and nurses involved in taking care of the patient. If we are all in agreement, then I discuss with the patient during rounds that day and prepare them for the timing of their discharge. ~*~

Then my OT comes back this last day, and this time she's got the walker and crutches both (for training me on), and is accompanied by my PT. Aha! They're ganging up on me! I suspect they are here together in case I am unable to navigate the stairs and they should need to catch me. She also got one of the many things she's been teaching me about—it's called a *sock puller* which she now shows me how to use (**See Figures 13.4 and 13.5**) and helps me get my socks on, and today I'm to get completely dressed as well. She shows me how to put my trousers on next and finally my tennis shoes—*my going home shoes*—woohoo! So, again, out we go to the stairwell, and I practice ascending and descending the stairs with my OT beside me and my PT behind me—but this time, even though they are there to catch me or intervene if needed—I have to do it all on my own. So, I go slowly and carefully, doing everything they've taught me to (while they coach and safeguard me all the way and I do just fine. We then go back to my room and my PT clears me to wander the halls as much as I want—without an escort—and all dressed up to go home. Wow! Then my last lunch comes and it's really good.

Note: your OT and PT may not do with you exactly what they did with me. Much of what goes on is dictated by your surgeon's preferences, how well you're doing, your age and strength, and a host of other variables.

In the afternoon here comes Dr. Hugate again. He's all smiles and has seen my reports, chart, and test results and spoken with all of my caregivers—and knows I'm ready to go home. He leaves and now comes the waiting.

190

Yep, I'm waiting for my wife to come and get me so we can go home.

The last day at the hospital is a trying, challenging time, a time of both great happiness and serious anticipation. There is a veritable blizzard of paperwork, approvals, and crosschecks, all to get me checked out and discharged. My PT and OT have given me a sheet of home instructions—lots of instructions. My floor nurse has given me another sheet of instructions. Dr. Hugate left home instructions and prescriptions, and there are the general discharge papers to sign. Essentially every person I've been working with has given me some written instructions to take home, I call all these my "marching orders." I have to be sure to take care of these papers and not lose them in the business of getting home too. They have instructions on everything from how to bathe from my PT and OT both, to Dr. Hugate's instructions about not getting the incision wet, and so on, and so forth.

Finally, when all the necessary discharge paperwork is ready, my floor nurse comes with a wheel chair, my wife gathers up all the stuff I've accumulated during my four day journey, and the caravan downstairs begins—my wife, my nurse and the transport staff guy—and me in a wheel chair (they always wheel you out, it's policy). Once we reach the big double glass doors, my wife goes on ahead and retrieves the car from the parking garage. Then I come to another of these first challenges: getting into a car with a full-leg splint on. I'm only glad nobody was there with a candid video cam. At last, I'm leaving the hospital with a brand new joint in my leg, lots of hopes and dreams, and more than a little bit of worry.

So as I close this chapter, let's talk about that worry. Essentially, I've been watched over and helped by a group of excellent professionals and caregivers. Up to this point, I have never been alone. I've had a call button to ask for help, and had all my needs taken care of. There was a bevy of highly trained physicians on-call twenty-four hours per day in case I had any complications. I had somebody bringing me my meals and any snacks that I wanted. Now—suddenly—I'm headed for home and I know that next week my wife will go back to work and I'll be all alone. Home alone? "Hey guys, can I just stay here a while longer?"

We have talked about this moment in other parts of our handbook. You have prepared your home, right? You have aligned your caregivers, correct? You are going back home and even though it is scary and challenging, you'll do fine. And thus ends this part of my story. I hope it serves you well in showing you a glimpse of the journey back to finding your new lease on life.

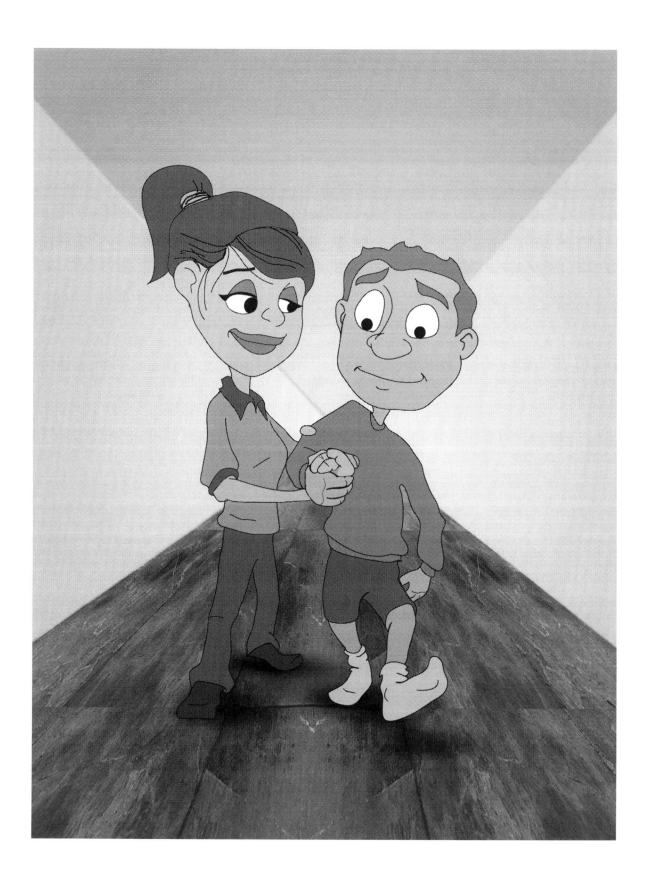

Physical Therapy for Hip and Knee Replacement Surgery

CHAPTER 14

by Inger Brueckner

Physical therapy is an important part of recovering from joint replacement. While the surgery removes and replaces the worn out surfaces of your joint, if you don't embark on an effort to get those parts moving and working again properly, you may be disappointed in the result. In this chapter, I'll use my 18 years experience as a Physical Therapist (PT) to give you a broad introduction to the subject. Let's start with a definition:

Physical therapy is a health profession involving the art and science of physical rehabilitation. Physical therapists work with patients by providing training, services, and assistance designed to maintain and/or restore maximum functional mobility for patients in whom movement and function have been compromised.

Hugate's Comment: Robert and I have repeatedly emphasized that undergoing successful knee or hip replacement surgery is only half the battle. Without good physical therapy following surgery, patients may fail to meet their goals. Physical therapists play many roles in your rehabilitation after joint replacement surgery. Trainer, instructor, motivator, friend, and advocate are just some of the many hats a physical therapist may wear. To get you better acquainted with who physical therapists are and what they do, we have invited Inger Brueckner MSPT, to describe the role of the PT and guide you through the process of functional recovery after joint replacement. Inger is a superb PT who specializes in rehabilitation following complex injuries and/or surgeries. ~*~

Here are some facts about PTs. In the USA, physical therapists must be licensed to practice, and to be licensed, they must graduate from an accredited program and also pass a national exam. When I became a physical therapist in the early 1990s, the training programs were in transition from an undergraduate (bachelor) degree to a Master of Science in Physical Therapy (MSPT) and these days, many universities offer a full doctorate. Most also advance their post-university education throughout their career by a combination of continuing education and specialized, extended training. Nowadays, PTs are considered primary care providers in many insurance networks and you can visit and seek treatment from a PT without a doctor's referral in most states. However, many insurance carriers (such as Medicare) will not cover physical therapy without a physician's prescription.

In addition, throughout the course of your physical therapy, you may also be treated by a *physical therapy assistant* (PTA) who works under the direct supervision of your PT. The PTA assists your PT in implementing your treatment plan. I'll speak more about your treatment plan later in this chapter.

Holland's Comment: *I dearly love physical therapists (and the therapy assistants too). Working as a team, they have many times given me back the life and mobility I had when I was younger. Of all the heroes on my medical team, they are the ones who give me the toughest love too. Sometimes the things they do, like massaging cramped muscles, putting cold packs on the knee, using electrical stimulation devices for pain reduction, and helping me stand up correctly, are painful—that is, they hurt when I'm doing it, but feel wonderful afterwards. They always seem to know what's best for me and—whether I'm stalling, whining, or being uncooperative—they know how to use stern words to chide me.*

Here's the thing: there is "bad pain," like how the knee throbbed in agony before the TKR every time I got home from the mall, a bicycle ride, or a hike; and there is "good pain," like the pain I have from healing up my new knee. So I just make up my mind that I will embrace the "pain of healing," and relish reclaiming my freedom and mobility. ~~*

Types of Physical Therapy

Over the course of recovery from joint replacement, you will see PTs in various settings. In this section, we will explore the two main types of physical therapy: inpatient (that is: physical therapy while you are in the hospital), and outpatient.

Inpatient Physical Therapy

The initial phase of physical therapy after joint replacement surgery involves the inpatient (in-hospital) PT. The inpatient PT's goals are different than the outpatient PT's goals. The inpatient PT's goal is to get you home as soon and safely as possible following surgery. This involves teaching you independence with the activities of daily living (ADLs). ADLs are those physical tasks which we perform every day at home, such as getting in and out of bed, bathing, using the toilet, walking in the house, preparing meals, and getting dressed. Mastery of the ADLs is a minimum basic requirement for discharge from the hospital.

The inpatient PT's job is to motivate you to do your best even when you are feeling ill, medicated, or in pain—to get you up and moving your new joint as soon as possible. Patients who mobilize quickly following joint replacement surgery have improved range of motion and less risk of bed-sores, blood clots, pneumonia, and other complications.

Outpatient Physical Therapy

Once you're discharged from the hospital, you'll work with the PT involved in the final (and most important) phase of rehabilitation known as the outpatient PT. You can usually choose the therapist you want to work with when in the outpatient setting. Many of Dr. Hugate's instructions in *Chapter 3, How to go about Finding a Surgeon: Do's and Don'ts* apply to selecting a PT as well. You can ask your surgeon, PCP, or someone you know who has gone through a joint replacement for their recommendations. Keep in mind you must find a physical therapy clinic which works with your insurance. It's also important to choose a physical therapy clinic in a convenient location, as you will be visiting often.

I always suggest that my patients:

Make arrangements for physical therapy before you go in for surgery.

When choosing a clinic, you should ask to take a tour. This would be a good opportunity to see if there are any other joint replacement patients at the clinic and get their opinion of the clinic. Outpatient PTs have a larger variety of equipment and treatment techniques at their disposal. In outpatient therapy, instead of only focusing on the ADLs, your PT will work on returning you to normal function and even recreational activities, such as golf.

Remember, no matter what the phase of physical therapy, you, the patient, are the most important ingredient of the rehabilitation process. The more involved you are, the better your outcome. If you don't know why you are working on a particular exercise, simply ask. Any competent and caring PT will welcome such questions and have logical and understandable answers at the ready. At times, it may seem like your PT will pick only those exercises for your rehabilitation plan that you find the most difficult. This is because those exercises which you find most difficult are most likely targeting the areas of your body that are weakest and most in need of work. If you're not challenged by an exercise, you're probably not working to your full potential.

I'd also like to take a moment here to talk about occupational therapists (OTs). OTs often work side-by-side with PTs. Their focus is to get you back to performing your everyday tasks independently. OTs may teach you how to get dressed, put your shoes on, pick an object up safely from the floor, get up from the floor if you have fallen, or how to safely get in or out of your car. They will also introduce you to several functional assistance devices such as the reacher/grabber (See Figure 14.1) and a long shoe-horn—all of which will help you return to independent function in everyday life. There is some overlap between physical therapy and occupational therapy, which is why these professionals are often found working together.

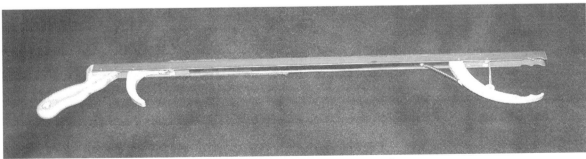

Figure 14.1 Photo of a generic grabber (reach extender device)

Initial (post-operative) Evaluation

When PTs first evaluate joint replacement patients, we look at a number of factors. We review the surgeon's prescription to verify the surgical site, type of surgery, and determine if there are any special requests or limitations. We then review medical history and baseline function, including baseline flexibility, strength, balance, and gait. We look at how well you get into and out of beds and chairs, and how you manage your ADLs in general. Next, through personal interactions, we explore your goals and desired levels of functionality and develop a customized treatment plan. This plan breaks down the steps necessary to meet your personal goals.

The relationship between patient and PT should be based on mutual trust and respect.

Your PT will likely push you past your comfort zone, working with you for the best possible outcome, and this requires that you do your part to help.

Doing your part involves respecting the limits we set for activities. Be diligent about performing your assigned exercises the exact number of times and in the manner instructed. Many patients think that doing more than they've been assigned is better. This can cause setbacks which actually extend the amount of days you'll be seeing the PT. It can also over-tax the surgical site, which has other implications, such as wound complications or excessive formation of scar tissue.

As part of the initial evaluation, we'll discuss the level of pain you're experiencing. Physical therapy can sometimes be painful. It is the pain from strengthening and healing which you must manage and tolerate now—during your recovery—that can help eliminate pain later on. Keep the lines of communication open and if one of the exercises causes you to experience significant pain let your PT know about it. We can sometimes make small adjustments to how you are performing an exercise and make it less painful.

It may be helpful to take pain medications before you come to therapy. Most of the stronger pain medications have driving restrictions when in use, so you have to plan on getting help with transportation to and from the therapy office. The medications can be very helpful but they won't take away all of the pain. They don't take effect right away either, so plan ahead. Most pain medications should be taken about thirty minutes prior to starting the physical therapy session.

By decreasing your pain, you can often decrease some of your muscle guarding. Muscle guarding occurs when you resist what your PT is trying to do for you, and

197

essentially work against the therapy because of the pain. Working through pain is a fine line to walk for both you and your therapist.

I've seen patients who, for whatever reason, did not follow through with physical therapy. This is a bad decision. Their motivation for this may be a lack of time, money, or transportation; not understanding how hard the process would be; or simply not making it a priority. These patients may reengage in physical therapy after they've stiffened up and make attempts to get their motion and function back—but this is sometimes not possible. If a replaced joint (especially knee) stiffens up, it may require further surgery to regain full and proper motion. If you're going to invest in having a joint replaced, make sure you get the most bang for your buck and find a way to get into physical therapy right after surgery.

If you have any financial difficulties, a physical therapy clinic can work with you concerning financial issues and get them settled before surgery. Physical Therapy clinics may know of resources available in the community and other strategies for a patient who has a difficult financial situation.

At this point, I'll describe a typical course of physical therapy—first for knee replacement, and then for hip replacement. Remember, this is a generic description of a routine postoperative course of therapy. Your situation may not be exactly the same, but will likely have many of these same elements.

Physical Therapy after Knee Replacement

Physical therapy is an especially important part of rehabilitation after knee replacement. Most physical therapy protocols allow a patient some time to recover from surgery with no active physical therapy on the day of surgery. Your in-hospital caregivers may use a continuous passive motion (CPM) machine (**See Figure 14.2**) to start with gentle flexing and extending the new knee joint.

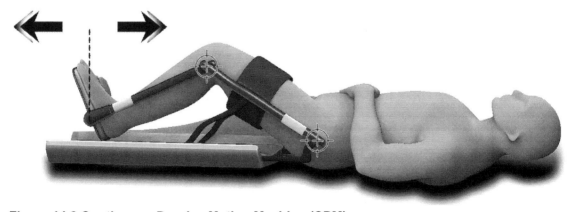

Figure 14.2 Continuous Passive Motion Machine (CPM)

198

The CPM is usually applied to the knee soon after surgery. Note that the CPM must be positioned correctly in order for you to reap the benefits. If the CPM is uncomfortable in spite of the pain medications, it may not be positioned correctly, or it may not be working properly. If this is the case, ask your nurse or PT to take a look at your CPM unit and ensure that it's positioned and adjusted appropriately.

As soon as the initial resting period following surgery is over, the inpatient PT will start helping you bend and straighten your knee. Obviously, if your doctor has ordered a CPM machine, this is already helping to get your new knee moving. However, while I personally believe that CPM machines have their place in TKR rehabilitation, I warn patients that the CPM will not give you all the motion your knee will need. The CPM is a simply an assistive tool, something to be used as a complement to—not instead of—physical therapy.

The work of mobilizing, transferring, and walking again begins shortly after surgery. In the days immediately after the operation, patients often see the inpatient PT at least twice daily for thirty to forty-five minutes per visit. The focus is on basic transfers, ambulation, ADLs, and simple motion/strength exercises. You'll also get a home program of exercises to start once you're discharged from the hospital.

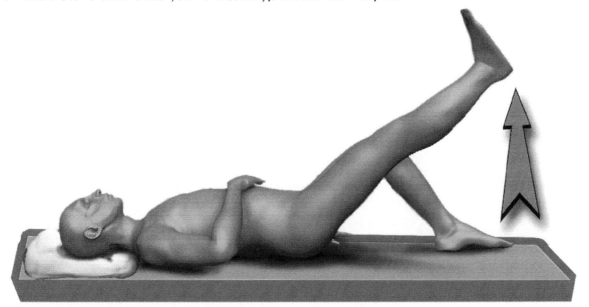

Figure 14.3 Illustration of Straight Leg Raise

The straight leg raise is one of the most basic exercises the inpatient PT starts with. Here, you simply raise your leg off the bed while keeping the knee straight. This simple activity strengthens the quadriceps muscles of the thigh and the flexors of the hip (**See Figure 14.3**).

Some patients can lift their leg, but are unable to keep the knee straight. This is called an extensor lag and is measured by the number of degrees that the knee remains bent while lifting the entire leg. The more the knee is unable to straighten, the worse the extensor lag (indicating weakness in the quadriceps muscles). If you have a significant extensor lag, a knee brace may be used to keep your leg straight and help protect your knee when your quadriceps muscles aren't strong. Doing a straight leg raise independently (without a knee brace) and being able to bend your knee very close to 90 degrees are two of the goals your PT wants you to meet before you leave the hospital.

The inpatient PT will also teach you how to get in and out of both a bed and a chair safely. Being at least independent with these transfers—which means that you don't need help from a caregiver for a specific activity—is another goal you should meet before discharge from the hospital.

The first day you're up, you may stand at the edge of the bed or even walk for a short distance around your room. On the second visit in the afternoon, you may be asked to walk to the door or the bathroom, and you may get to sit in a chair. These activities are expanded upon in the second and third day until you are able to walk down the hall. With each physical therapy session, you'll be asked to go farther. The goal with these exercises is for you to be able to walk 150 to 200 feet and manage stairs safely before discharge.

Back at Home after Knee Replacement

Once you are discharged from the hospital, you will begin the outpatient phase of physical therapy. Some people have difficulty in getting to an outpatient clinic to continue therapy immediately after discharge from the hospital. In these cases, at-home physical therapy, in which a PT comes to your home, may be the best option for filling that gap until you are able to make it to the therapy clinic. The availability of at-home physical therapy depends on your needs, finances, and insurance. The at-home therapists can analyze the issues you're dealing with at home and help find strategies to overcome those issues. If you receive at-home physical therapy, the PT will typically come as often as two to three times per week at the beginning of your treatment.

A drawback of at-home physical therapy is that they seldom have access to the equipment found in a typical outpatient therapy clinic. It's a lot easier for a PT to work on your balance, move a stiff knee, or manage the progress of even the more able patients when all of the tools of the trade are at hand.

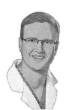

Hugate's Comment: *Do yourself a favor and make arrangements in advance of your surgery to have someone help you get to and from the physical therapy clinic after surgery. At-home PTs are limited in the options available to help you rehabilitate because they must tote all of their equipment around with them. As soon as you are safely able, plan to go to the physical therapy clinic and have your therapy sessions done there. ~*~*

Remember, although the majority of patients are able to go home after surgery, if you've had any complications, don't meet the minimum physical therapy requirements, or have other serious underlying medical difficulties, you may need to go to a rehabilitation facility, or an extended care facility instead of going home from the hospital immediately. At these other venues you'll have a PT and continue to progress toward your mobility until you can go home safely.

Typically, your doctor will order outpatient physical therapy two to three times per week for six to eight weeks after knee replacement. A standard treatment session in the outpatient physical therapy clinic might start out with a warm-up on an upright stationary bike. You'll likely not be able to complete a full revolution on the bike pedals initially because you won't have the range of motion yet. So first, your PT will have you do three-quarter revolutions on the pedals and keep working at it from there. She'll have you go backward and forward with the pedals, stretching each way as you go, until you're able to go all the way around. You can usually complete a full revolution on the bicycle pedals when you're able to comfortably bend your knee to about 100 degrees of flexion. As time goes on, she might lower the seat on the bike, which forces you to bend the knee even further to complete a full revolution.

Next, we begin with "passive stretching". This is where you simply lie there and your PT does the work of stretching for you (**See Figure 14.4**). She starts by straightening your knee, which she does by pushing downward on the knee while you're lying flat on your back. She then works on bending the knee by

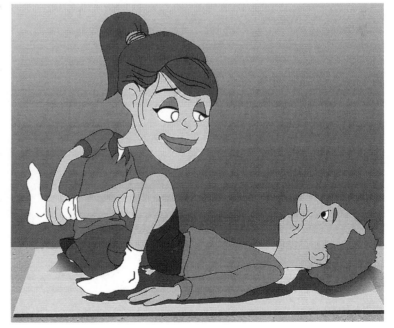

Figure 14.4 Cartoon of PT administering passive stretching

201

doing the opposite, which is to push your ankle toward your buttocks. Then, she'll turn you over and position you lying on your stomach. Once you're lying face down, she'll stretch your quadriceps and hamstrings by going through similar motions again.

Then it's on to the parallel bars (**See Figure 14.5**) to stand on a balance board and do some step-ups. Step-ups are where you step up onto (and back down off of) a slightly elevated platform. The parallel bars are used to maintain balance during the exercise. Next, while you're still there, she'll work on improving your walking (known as your gait). She analyzes and decomposes your gait into small components and has you practice them one or two at a time while she watches and systematically cues you into walking correctly.

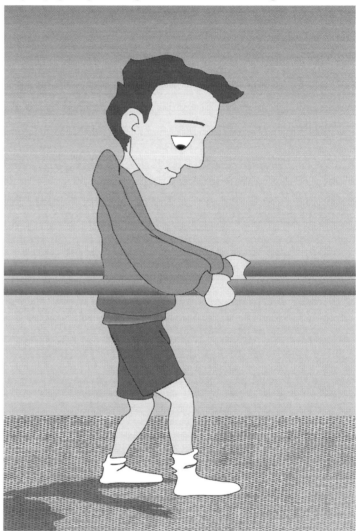

Figure 14.5 Cartoon of patient using parallel bars for stability

Holland's Comment:

 A person's gait is how they walk — or, in my case, limp before having my TKR. There are at least thirteen different types of gait. The one I developed the bad habit of using is known as an "antalgic gait", meaning that I limped in such a manner as to reduce pain on weight-bearing structures in my knee. Before I had the TKR, I thought I was strong and tough. It turned out that I had been protecting (or favoring) my right knee for many years. The result was that my buttock muscles were very weak. After my TKRs, my PT had to reeducate me in how to place my feet, lift my legs, step forward, and stand up straight while walking. Over the course of my physical therapy, with loving care, and constant admonitions, I essentially learned to walk correctly from scratch.

202

Another issue we discovered after my first TKR was that my PT was initially focusing her therapeutic efforts on the surgical site only—namely my knee. I explained that I was experiencing increasing pain in my lower back and neck. It was then that we realized I was creating an imbalance by working only the operative leg. We then began strengthening my buttocks, abdomen, and lower back as well and it was only after these increased efforts on all of the muscles affected by debilitating pain in the old knee joint that my recovery took a turn for the better. As my gait improved, the pain in my lower back and neck slowly disappeared as well. ~*~

Typically, some sort of sliding back-board is next. You lie down on a board and push against resistance. There are a number of different kinds, some use various springs which your PT can engage for varying degrees of resistance. Others (**See Figure 14.6**) are simply padded boards that travel on rails using your own weight as resistance. This exercise strengthens all of your thigh and leg muscles working them all in both directions—alternately contracting and relaxing—helping re-establish coordination between antagonistic muscle groups. The idea is to extend your operative leg (using the extensor mechanism) and then flex your leg under tension (using the hamstrings), thus, increasing strength and flexibility in both directions.

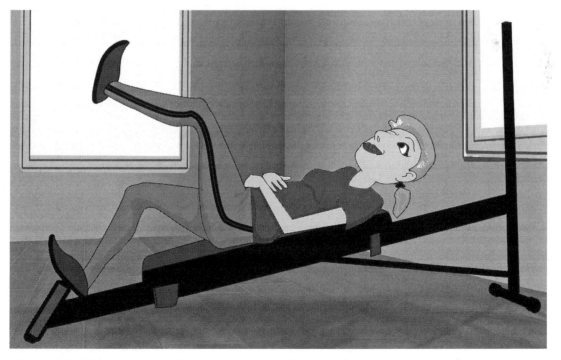

Figure 14.6 Cartoon of a lady on a sliding backboard strengthening her operative leg

Now, your PT may have you lean against the (See Figure 14.7). Exercises requiring you to move your non-operative leg while exercising with your operative leg are also excellent. All of these exercises can be modified to become steadily harder and more challenging each week. Your PT will accomplish this by increasing both repetitions and resistance.

Last, your PT will usually mobilize your scar. This is a form of massage used to break up scar tissue under your incision and improve pain and motion. You see, scar tissue starts forming shortly after surgery and may bind up the knee and make the knee overly sensitive. Mobilizing this tissue allows the extensor mechanism to glide under the skin rather than being 'stuck to' the skin and stiffening up.

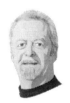 **Holland's Comment:** *Once you have permission from your surgeon, you can do this for yourself at home. Scar mobilization can be challenging in the moment, but after you've done the work there's a great deal of relief. This is another one of those "good pains" I talk about. You can also employ the use of some sort of lubricant like hand lotion, massage cream, or massage oil. Your local pharmacy has various specialized ointments for scar massage, simply ask your pharmacist. ~*~*

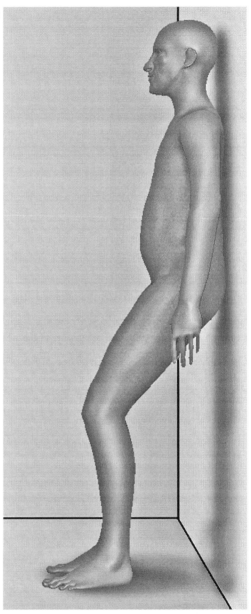

Figure 14.7 Balance Assisted Squat

After each day's session, your PT will typically ice your knee while you rest and relax a bit (and sometimes even use electro-stimulation), all to keep the exercises and work you've done from causing unacceptable pain and/or swelling.

Most of my patients understand how important regaining knee flexion (bending) is. They need adequate bending to get in and out of the car, sit comfortably in a chair, and even to get dressed.

However, our biggest concern is this:

You must restore your knee's straightening as soon as possible.

I prefer that my patients have full knee extension before they see me in the outpatient setting, but that does not always happen. There seems to be a small window of four to six weeks after surgery in which to get the knee straight. After that crucial period, it gets progressively more difficult and more painful to work on straightening. If your knee doesn't get fully straight during this critical period, your PT will spend extra time trying to get the knee to straighten.

Holland's Comment: When I was in therapy with my own PT, she had me buy a set of strap-on weights consisting of a pouch with hook-and-loop straps, and pockets on the outside into which are placed small weights. This small assembly then wraps around your ankle (or can be hung from your knee when sitting) to provide resistance. These can be purchased at almost any sporting goods or athletic store. The weight of the unit could be adjusted from two ounces all the way to two pounds. With these weights, I was able to perform a number of helpful exercises. I'll describe several of the most important uses for these little, ankle weights.

During that first six weeks after surgery, every night while watching TV, I sat in my chair with a thick pillow on a low bench under my operative leg's heel and put the little weight pack across my knee until it became uncomfortable (See Figure 14.8). Then I'd take it off and wait a while, then go for it again. I started out with a few of the little

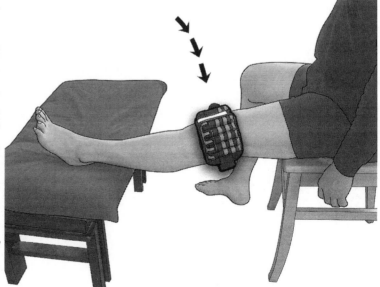

Figure 14.8 Illustration showing ankle weights being used to help straighten the operative knee

weights and when that no longer hurt after about fifteen minutes in place, on the next night I added two or three more of the two-ounce weights. After about three weeks, I could tolerate the entire two pounds—but still could not fully straighten my operative leg. Then, during the next three weeks I kept at it—and kept at it—and as every night went by I could stand the two-pound ankle-weight hanging on my knee a little bit longer. Every day I noticed I could also straighten my leg a tiny bit more.

The rest of these passive stretches use gravity and weights as well. While sitting in a chair, I would strap the weights around my ankle and hold my operative leg out straight to strengthen my thigh muscles. Another one I did (with the weights still strapped to my ankle) was to lay on the edge of the bed—on my stomach with my legs hanging over—and allow the operative leg to simply hang there. The weights on my ankle acted to pull the knee into a straight position. This can be done without weights too and is far more challenging than you'd think. When I had my post-operative exam six weeks after surgery, I was able to get my leg to a tiny bit past 0 degrees.~*~

When your knee is swollen, or won't straighten comfortably, you'll want to keep a pillow or towel roll under it, to make it more comfortable. Resist the urge! You can use this position for a short time to gain relief, but if you keep something under your knee, it will become accustomed to being in a bent position and heal in this bent position. If you sleep or sit with a pillow under the knee, it will become more and more difficult and painful to straighten it. Try to strike a balance. Getting a full, restful night of sleep is vital for healing, but if you can't sleep without a pillow under your knee, you'll have to work that much harder during the day to straighten it. For this reason you should try to get your leg into a position where it tries to become straight every chance you get—be committed and determined.

Hugate's Comment: I strongly discourage any patient who is healing from knee replacement surgery from putting anything under the knee itself for the same reasons Inger provides. If the knee is uncomfortable when you're working on full extension in whatever setting, I recommend that you use pain medications. If those aren't adequate, call your surgeon's office and maybe try some other pain medication until you find a combination that works. ~*~

What if, despite all this physical therapy, your motion does not return? Fortunately this is rare, but there are a few options. If the knee joint gets to a certain amount of bending and then hits a "brick wall" and won't go any further, you may have thick scar tissue and may need to undergo a procedure called manipulation under anesthesia (MUA). This is a procedure in which you go to sleep for a few minutes in the operating room while the surgeon moves the knee back and forth, breaking up the scar tissue. Because you're asleep, there is no immediate pain, though the knee will of course be sore after an MUA. If you undergo an MUA, your PT will usually see you daily for two weeks afterward to help maintain the range of motion accomplished. This is a very effective technique but does cause pain and sometimes bruising.

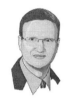 **Hugate's Comment:** I reserve MUA as a last-resort option. Inger describes the procedure well, and as she notes, it is rare that we need to perform an MUA. This is generally a decision that I will make with feedback from the patient and the PT as to how thick and tenacious the scar tissue is. The daily physical therapy for two weeks following an MUA that Inger refers to is a redoubling of efforts to help ensure that the scar tissue doesn't simply return putting you back to square one.

If the scar tissue is not quite as thick, your PT (after discussion with your surgeon) may try braces or splints to achieve the motion necessary, along with aggressive physical therapy. In general, PTs don't tend to use much splinting except for the knee immobilizer early on for an extension stretch. But in an especially difficult knee, we will use these aids. If you have a neuropathy (numbness in the leg or feet), diabetes, or vascular problems (poor circulation), be sure to let your PT know, as this will affect how tightly a splint or brace can be mounted on your leg. ~*~

Every patient is different, and even each knee on the same patient is different (in the case of bilateral knee replacements). I've had very difficult knees to treat, and very easy ones. Some patients experience so much relief from the surgery that the rehabilitation to regain range of motion and strength is very easy. Physical therapy on your knee will require hard work and persistence, but you can rest assured that your efforts will pay off in much improved strength and mobility in the long run.

Physical Therapy after Hip Replacement

Physical therapy for hip replacement is going through some big changes as we write this handbook. There are different surgical approaches, different types of hip replacements, and minimally invasive techniques that affect what kind of therapy your orthopedic surgeon orders for rehabilitation. All of these variables change what type of physical therapy you receive in the hospital and during outpatient rehabilitation as well. Next, we will go over the typical postoperative rehabilitation course after total hip replacement.

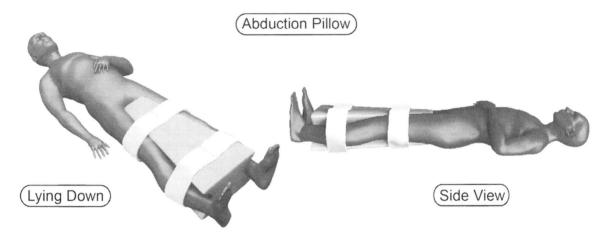

Figure 14.9 Illustration of patient in abduction pillow

Surgeons will sometimes use a special pillow called an abduction pillow for their patients after hip replacement surgery. An abduction pillow is a triangular, foam pillow that is placed between your legs immediately after surgery to keep you from crossing your legs (**See Figure 14.10**). Crossing your legs right after hip replacement surgery is discouraged, as it can lead to dislocation of the new hip replacement. Above (**See Figure 14.9**) is an illustration of a patient strapped into an

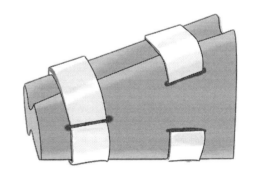

Figure 14.10 Illustration of abduction pillow

abduction pillow as it would be used in the hospital or at home. Please note that this pillow is never used standing up. Also note that the risk of dislocation goes down over time and most surgeons generally don't require a hip abduction pillow to be used beyond a few days unless there are extenuating circumstances.

You will also be instructed in "ankle pump" exercises (**See Figure 14.11**). You will perform these every hour while you are awake in the hospital for the first few days after your surgery to aid the blood circulation in your leg. The ankle pump exercise is very simple. For the first part of this exercise, you straighten out your foot, pointing your toes away from your body as best you can. For the second half of the ankle pump, you bend your foot and try to point your toes at your head. Wiggling your toes is good too. Repeat this at least ten times whenever you do it.

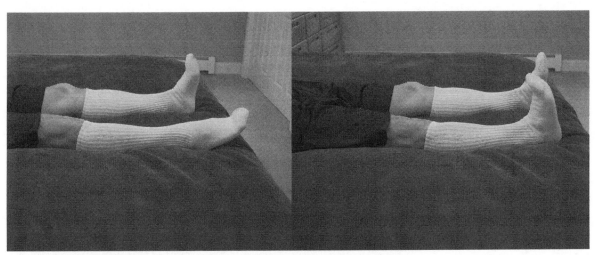

Figure 14.11 Photo of a patient doing ankle pumps with right leg

The most common hip replacement approach is the posterior approach (curved incision along the back of the buttock). The information in this chapter will therefore focus on rehabilitation for that approach. If your surgeon uses a different approach, their recommendations would be somewhat different.

Early on, you will learn from your physical therapist about the so-called "hip precautions." One of the potential complications after hip replacement surgery is that of dislocation (the new hip popping out of its socket). This is rare, but the risk for dislocation is highest in the early days and weeks following hip replacement surgery. The hip precautions are a set of rules which dictate that you keep your hips out of certain positions that put them at risk for dislocating. The hip precautions will differ slightly depending on the technique that your surgeon uses to install the hip. This list of rules should be written down for you, and you should commit them to memory. It's best to also have a family member or close friend write these rules down and remember them so they can help you follow the hip precautions after surgery. The most common reason that people dislocate their hips after joint replacement surgery is failure to follow the hip precautions. So, I'll take some time here to go through each of the hip precautions associated with the posterior hip approach.

Hip Precaution #1, Don't bend your hip beyond 90 degrees.

You must avoid any seated position which makes your knees higher than your hips.

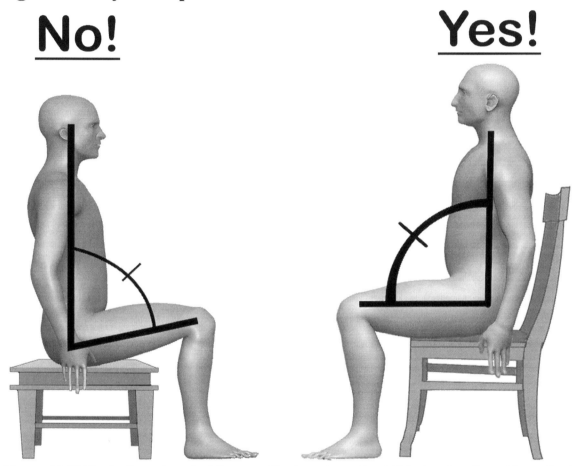

No!   **Yes!**

Figure 14.12 Illustration of seated figures: The bench on the left is too low for a hip patient. Note that the knees are ABOVE the hips. The chair on the right is just high enough for a hip patient. Note that the knees are EVEN with hips.

     The angle between your body and your operative hip should never be less than 90 degrees. There are several ways people (inadvertently) break this rule. First, let's look at sitting down. If you sit on an object that is too low, your hip will bend too much. (**See Figure 14.12**).You must avoid any seated position which makes your knees higher than your hips and remember to be very cautious when standing from a seated position.

I encourage my patients to install toilet seat extenders (**See Figure 14.13**). Not only does it make your commode more comfortable to sit on, it helps you maintain hip precautions and is much easier on you when standing back up. With a generic toilet seat extender like the one on the left you're a lot less likely to need help in the bathroom. Also be cognizant that it's very easy to inadvertently lean too far forward when regaining your feet.

Lastly, remember that in most homes and public restrooms those toilet seats are too low as well. With this in mind—and for your own safety—make it a habit to use the handicap stall complete with grab bars and an ADA-compliant commode while you are rehabilitating.

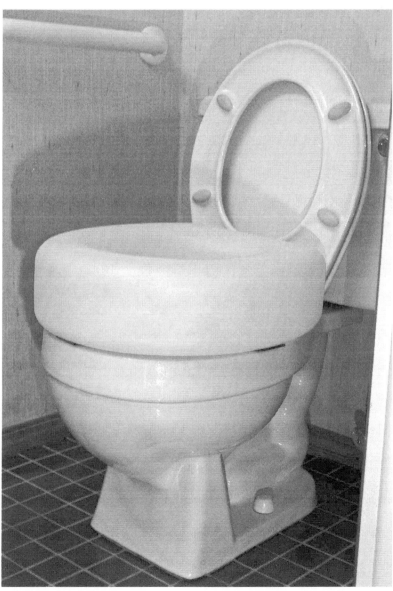

Figure 14.13 Photo of a non-ADA commode with toilet seat extender

Another way that this rule is broken inadvertently is while picking up objects off of the floor. If you bend forward at the hips and pick an object up directly from the floor you will flex the hip too much (**See figure 14.14**).

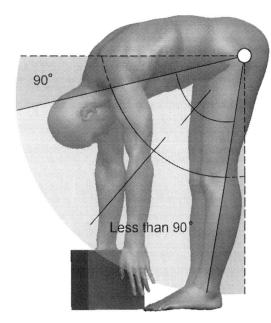

A good rule of thumb for bending down is this—if your hand is lower than your knees, you've bent down too far.

Instead, try these other two strategies for picking objects from the floor as shown on the right and below (**See Figures 14.15 and 14.16**).

Figure 14.14 Illustration of <u>incorrect</u> way to bend down and pick up an object

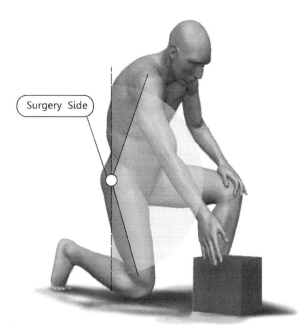

Figure 14.15 Illustration of a safe strategy for picking an object up by kneeling

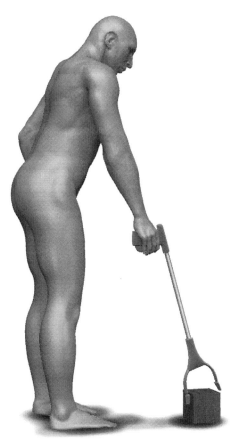

Figure 14.16 Illustration of a safe strategy for picking an object up using a grabber.

212

Hip Precaution #2—Do not cross your legs.

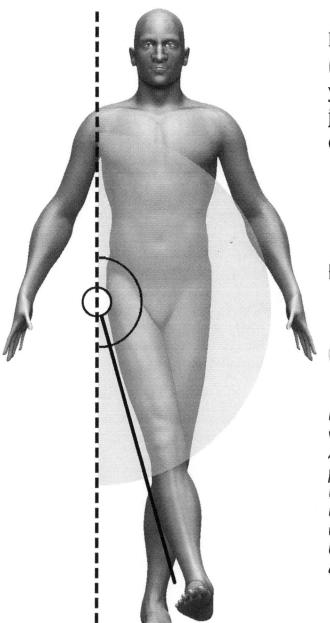

Extreme crossing of the legs (See Figure 14.17) can pop your hip replacement out of joint, especially in the early days after hip replacement.

Hugate's Comment:

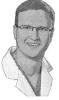

While this rule is self-explanatory, it can be quite difficult to track when sleeping. Many patients (especially those who sleep on their side) inadvertently cross their legs while trying to get comfortable. At least initially, the abductor pillow will help alleviate this issue. For this reason, it's safest during initial recovery period after hip replacement to sleep on your back. It's a lot less likely that you'll accidently cross your legs. ~*~

Figure 14.17 Illustration of unstable hip position after hip replacement (legs crossed). Avoid this position

Hip Precaution #3—Do not turn your toes inward.

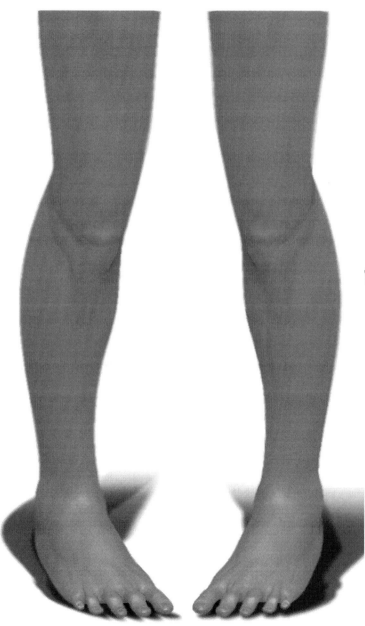

Figure 14.18 Illustration of unstable hip position after hip replacement (toes turned inward). Avoid this position.

Keep your toes pointing straight ahead or slightly outward (See Figure 14.18).

Hugate's Comment:

This means not to rotate your leg such that your toes are pointing inward. This is usually the easiest of the three rules to follow. It's rare that you turn your toes inward during your every day routine. However, on occasion, you'll sometimes turn your feet inward when you abruptly change direction. Your PT and OT will both teach you ways to make your turns without having to rotate your foot excessively. ~*~

During your hospital stay, both the PT and OT will teach you about (and help remind you of) the hip precautions specific to your surgery. Soon these rules will become second nature, but for the first few days after surgery, you

214

should have these cautious reminders easily at hand. It's a good idea to have them posted somewhere in your room so you can be constantly reminded of them. The PT and OT will also teach you strategies for performing everyday tasks without breaking the hip precaution rules. You will need to practice how to get your clothes on while not being able to bend over excessively at the waist. The OT will issue you special pieces of equipment, like a reacher, extended shoe-horn, and a sock-aid that'll help you avoid bending over at the hip while getting your socks and shoes on. It's also best to consider putting aside your lace-up shoes and bringing slip-on shoes to the hospital; these are much easier and safer to use after hip replacement because you don't have to bend over to get them on your feet.

Hugate's Comment: The hip precautions are important to know and live, especially for the first three months after surgery, when your hip is at the highest risk for dislocation. After that period, a thick capsule forms around the hip and your risk for dislocation goes down. It does not go down to zero, however, and most surgeons (including me) ask that their patients continue with the hip precautions to reduce their risk of ever dislocating the hip replacement in the future. Don't worry—soon these precautions become second nature.

If you ever feel your hip is in an unstable position, then stop what you are doing and move to a position of safety. Your hip is more stable (less likely to dislocate) if you keep your knees apart, stand straight up, and point your toes forward. Keep this safe-position in mind and slowly move to that position if you feel you're at risk for dislocating the hip.

As Inger mentioned, we are here describing the standard precautions after the most common type of hip approach, the posterior approach. Be sure and communicate with your surgeon and PT to find out what specific precautions they would like you to follow after your surgery. ~*~

Each day you're in the hospital (starting the day after surgery), you'll be given leg-strengthening exercises and instructed on how to move in bed and stand up following your precautions for weight bearing status. Unlike physical therapy for knee replacement patients, physical therapy for hip replacement patients focuses on ADLs, early ambulation, and weight bearing. Unless there is an unusual circumstance, your surgeon typically allows you to put full weight on the hip replacement immediately after surgery.If you are prescribed at-home physical therapy, you will be seen a few times to ensure you are safe and independent at home. The at-home PT and OT will also help you increase strength and ambulation through a series of simple exercises mostly focused on strengthening your

215

gluteal (buttock) muscles. Getting in and out of your car, as well as up and off of the floor (if you fall) can be tricky tasks for the first days and weeks after surgery. After a hip replacement, your pain, hip strength, or the hip precautions, may limit your choices on how to go about these tasks safely.

Once you are able to start at an outpatient physical therapy clinic, your surgeon will generally order physical therapy for two times a week for two to four weeks. Most hip replacement patients will run through a progression similar to that of knee replacement patients.

Your PT will start by having you warm up your legs with a gentle aerobic activity where the type of exercise varies depending on your particular circumstances. Then, she'll work on stretching if you have any flexibility issues. With a hip replacement patient, a PT will spend more time on balance and balance reactions than with a knee patient. If you have been unable to put all of your weight through your hip, it is very important to work on these activities. She'll start weight bearing advancement first with the use of parallel bars as a safety aid and then advance to walking without a walker or crutches.

The most common problem that hip replacement patients encounter during rehabilitation is gluteal (buttock muscle) weakness, especially the muscle called the "gluteus medius" or "hip abductor" (**See Figure 14.19**) This results in a characteristic limp. Once you are allowed *full weight bearing* on the hip, it is important to strengthen these muscles on both sides (**See Figure 14.21**). It will make all the difference in how well you walk. Many hip replacement patients with a persistent limp can develop back pain, so it's important to expedite the strengthening of this muscle group to avoid the gait abnormalities and pains that may follow.

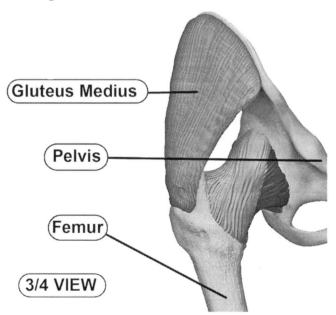

Figure 14.19 Illustration of the gluteus medius muscle from the right front side.

If you have a limp initially after surgery, don't be discouraged—this is common. At first, your PT will almost always have you using an assistive device to help ambulate safely until the weak gluteus muscle can be strengthened. Be assured she will choose a device that's the safest for your situation while still allowing you the most freedom.

Often we see a hip replacement patient who tries to stop using the cane too quickly. If your gluteal muscles aren't strong enough to hold you upright correctly (and support a proper gait), you will limp—and maybe even fall (**See Figure 14.20**). Remember, it can take a few weeks (and possibly longer), and a lot of hard work to restore your strength to a good baseline.

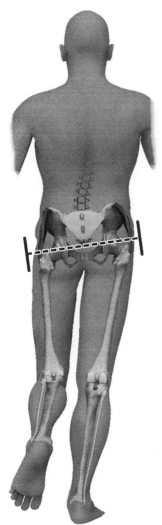

Figure 14.20
Illustration showing a weak gluteus medius and the resulting pelvic tilt with mis- alignment of the lower spine.

Holland's Comment:

Take it from me, having a weak gluteus medius causes your pelvis to tilt with each step you take and inevitably causes lower back pain. After both of my TKRs I had to work through my own lower-back pain issues. I lost count of how many times my PT patiently reassured me that my lower back would eventually stop hurting all the time—once I had strengthened these critical muscles and regained a normal gait.

In the illustration to the upper left (*Figure 14.20*), the right hip—as the figure is walking away—has a weak gluteus medius muscle. This allows the pelvis to tilt down-ward (toward the left side) when-ever the left leg is lifted during the ordinary processes of walking. The resulting limp and abnormal tilt of the pelvis, forces the lower back to compensate by curving back upward (to the right) so the person walking can remain bal-anced and not fall over. This cur-vature of the lower spine translates up through your spine all the way to your neck—affecting your entire back—but especially the lumbar region of your lower back. This imbalance in your gait eventually takes a toll

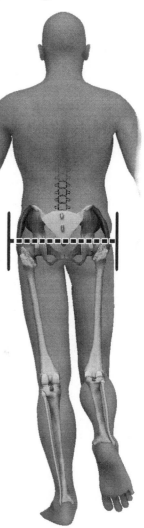

Figure 14.21
Illustration showing strong gluteus medius muscles properly sup- porting the pelvis and lower spine.

on your entire body—it did mine. This is the one of the reasons we stress physical therapy, guided strength exercises, and learning to walk without a limp throughout this handbook. ~*~

If you develop a persistent and severe limp, experience significant pain with any standing exercises, or are too weak to tolerate the gym exercises, then pool therapy may be an option for you. Generally speaking, you won't be swimming with this kind of therapy. Instead, you'll be performing exercises while in water that is at about your chest level. The water is heated slightly to improve your comfort and flexibility. The water both reduces your effective weight and adds gentle resistance to each movement during your exercises. This off-loads your joints and, for many people, can facilitate more effective physical therapy. However, you can't start pool therapy until your surgeon gives you their permission to submerge the incision. Also, there are some patients who shouldn't perform pool therapy. In general, if you have uncontrolled high blood pressure, seizure disorder, or an open wound, you probably won't be allowed to employ this particular form of physical therapy.

Be aware that insurance companies have decreased their coverage benefits for physical therapy over the years. This is something that we both (patient and PT) must be aware of because it may limit your access to therapy. Some plans allow only 10-15 visits to a PT per calendar year. Unfortunately, this means we have to put more and more responsibility back on you (as the patient) to follow through with exercises at home.

During your course of therapy, your PT will keep documentation on your progress (for a number of reasons) and will send your surgeon timely progress reports. If there are any concerns they will contact your surgeon. Orthopedic surgeons are busy people, so it can be hard to contact them. Your PT will help facilitate communication. It's much better to have the doctor see you when there's a small, manageable problem than to wait and let it become a serious issue.

In my practice, if I feel strongly that you need to be seen, I will be quite persistent with the office staff at the doctor's office. I'm used to making a nuisance of myself for my patient's sake. Some of the reasons I will contact your surgeon include:

- ***No progress made on your range of motion over four visits.***

- ***Lack of progress that cannot be explained.***

- ***Increased pain, redness, or swelling in your leg.***

218

- *If there are any concern about your incision.*

- *If your pain suddenly worsens.*

- *If you have a significant change in your sensation, balance, or strength.*

Hugate's Comment: One of the reasons that I think Inger is an excellent PT is her ability to get my attention when she feels one of my patients is "off-track." This is exactly the type of persistence and patient advocacy you want from your PT. As the old saying goes, "the squeaky wheel gets the grease." If your PT feels strongly that there is something wrong, it's important that she help get you where you need to be to have that issue addressed. ~*~

If everything is going fine, when you start getting close to your goals, I will decrease the number of times you come in per week, and then give you a two to four week period of time on your own. After that period, I have you come in for one final home program evaluation. The purpose of this visit is to make sure that you have a thorough home exercise program and it addresses all the areas you may still need work on after your outpatient physical therapy is complete.

Summary for PT

It's been my pleasure walking you through the processes of physical therapy, and rehabilitation after hip and knee replacement surgery. Getting your new joint going takes some dedication and hard work. Your PTs are there to help you along the way. We will get you up out of bed, back to your home, and then back to the activities you love to do. With this description of the process, you should be able to get yourself in the right mindset. The process is so much less intimidating if you know what to expect. Please remember to consider your relationship with your physical therapist a partnership and keep the lines of communication open.

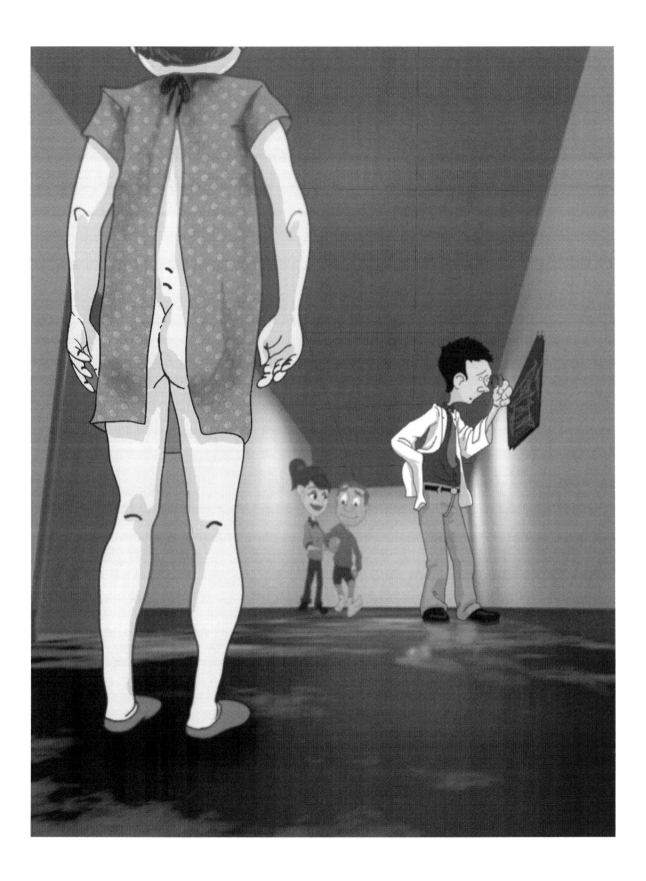

What Can Go Wrong?

CHAPTER 15

by Dr. Hugate

Although having a joint replacement has become routine in developed countries, it is still not without risk. Fortunately the vast majority of patients do well without major complications. But there are some potential problems, and this chapter of our handbook is dedicated to discussing those issues. Having this information is another important part of making your decision. You can't make an *informed choice* about whether to have surgery unless you know about both the risks and benefits of the procedure. Some of the risks we will discuss are more controllable than others.

It's important to realize that—while you should be made aware of the risks associated with joint replacement surgery—you could become overwhelmed with a discussion of each and every potential problem that may be encountered. For this reason, I will only discuss the *common* risks associated with joint replacement surgery. In addition, this chapter does not cover the topic of risk associated with anesthesia. My good friend and colleague, Dr. Gianni Checa, writes comprehensively about these risks in **Chapter 9, Anesthesia Options in Joint Replacement Surgery**. Where possible, I will try to give you a feeling for how common these issues may be—including statistics where available. Moreover, for balance, I will also cover preventive measures.

Bleeding

Bleeding is the first risk I usually discuss with patients. There will be some bleeding (of course) when you have surgery. There is typically a bit more blood loss during hip replacement surgery because of the depth of the hip joint (the amount of muscle and tissue around the hip joint) and the fact that we cannot use a tourniquet during hip replacement surgery. In the case of knee replacement surgery, most surgeons use a tourniquet on the thigh during the surgery so there is little or no blood loss during the actual surgery. A tourniquet is a pneumatic band that is wrapped around the thigh and inflated to a given pressure. The tourniquet compresses the thigh and does not allow blood to flow into the knee or leg during the surgery. This reduces blood loss and also makes it easier for the surgeon to see what he is doing. Of course when the surgery is complete, the tourniquet is deflated and the bleeding begins. Many surgeons place a drain inside the knee or hip to collect any blood that may accumulate there after surgery.

If there is substantial bleeding during or after surgery, it is possible that you may need a transfusion. A transfusion is a procedure where you are given blood (or components of blood) through an IV to replenish your supply. This is considered only when your blood count gets low enough to affect you. For example, if you become light-headed or dizzy, if your blood pressure is low, or your heart rate is high with a low blood count, we generally consider transfusion. We check the blood count daily, after surgery. We also have a lower threshold for transfusion in those with heart problems (because the heart relies on blood cells to deliver it oxygen). The risk for needing a transfusion after hip or knee replacement surgery varies from institution to institution and even between surgeons, but it can be generally estimated at about 10 to 30 percent.

Your risk for bleeding can be increased by a few other factors. If you are on blood thinners before surgery (such as anti-inflammatories, vitamin E, aspirin, or Coumadin) you may be at increased risk. If you're on any of these blood thinners, let your surgeon know well in advance of surgery so they can be managed before, during, and after surgery. There are also some medical conditions that increase the risk for bleeding. If you have a history of bruising easily, blood in your stool or urine, or heavy menstruation, let your doctor know before scheduling surgery.

If you need a transfusion, there are generally two options. Most patients receive blood from a blood bank. Blood banks (such as Red Cross or Bonfils) screen their blood donors and their donations very carefully to minimize the risk of transmitting disease. The risk for viral infection from transfusion is very, very low these days. According to the Red Cross, the current risk for transmitting HIV (the virus that causes AIDS) in a unit of blood transfused is about 1 in 2 million units; for acquiring hepatitis B is 1 in 200,000—500,000 units; and for acquiring hepatitis C is 1 in 1.39 million units. Another possible problem with blood transfusion is if you receive the incorrect blood type. There are extensive and redundant measures in place to prevent this from happening. The risk of getting the incorrect blood type in the United States is currently unknown because it is not routinely reported by medical facilities. But it is very, very rare—I have never seen it happen in my career. If this were to occur, however, it is unlikely that it would be fatal, but it would require medical treatment and close monitoring.

Some people prefer to place their own blood into the blood bank prior to surgery so that they can get it back if necessary after surgery. That is an acceptable plan, but the problem here is that you need to donate your blood within about thirty days before your surgery. Naturally, if you donate blood, your blood count will go down and you will enter into the surgery with a low blood count. This will (ironically) *increase* your risk for needing a transfusion because your starting blood level is low. So I do not insist that my patients auto-donate blood. There are also canister systems available that actually take your blood that is collected by the drain in your wound after surgery, store it, and allow it to be re-infused into your blood stream during your hospital stay. These systems are becoming more common, and they generally eliminate the issues with virus transmission and wrong blood type transfusions.

It's important to realize that should you need a transfusion, you will be made aware ahead of time of the possibility and will give consent for this to occur. There are patients who refuse transfusions—that is your right as a patient. If this is the case, please discuss with your surgeon well in advance so alternative strategies can be put in place to reduce your risk for transfusion even further.

Unwanted Blood Clots

Another risk of surgery is the exact opposite of bleeding: formation of unwanted blood clots. Of course, blood clotting is normal and necessary for bleeding to stop within the wound itself, but it is the clots that form *elsewhere* that can be problematic. For example, if a blood clot forms in the deep veins of your leg (the veins in the center of your leg), this is referred to as a deep venous thrombus (DVT). A DVT can cause problems with pain and swelling in the leg because it does not allow blood to flow effectively back to the body from the knee and lower leg.

An even more serious situation is when a DVT makes its way through the large veins and into the lungs. This is called a pulmonary embolism (or PE). Depending on the size, a PE can be fatal. If the clot is large it can "plug up" the lung and not allow oxygen into the blood. Fortunately, this is very rare. The risk of getting a DVT or PE depends on a number of factors. Overall risk of DVT in the USA is about 30 percent after knee replacement surgery and slightly lower after hip replacement. Most are extremely small, however, and go unnoticed. Only on rare occasions are DVTs big enough to be noticeable by the doctor or the patient. The risk of getting a PE is about 0.4 percent. Fortunately, the risk of fatality from PE is exceedingly low, less than 0.1 percent. There are clotting disorders that can cause clots and this would increase your risk for DVT or PE as well. If you have ever had a DVT or PE, or if you have an immediate family member who has, be sure and mention this to your doctor well in advance of surgery.

This discussion gives you special insight into one of the difficult and controversial areas of treatment after joint replacement surgery. We *want* you to form clots in your wound to prevent excessive bleeding and the need for blood transfusion, but we *don't want* you to form unwanted clots in your large, deep veins. We want your blood just thin enough to prevent DVT and PE but not so thin that it causes excessive bleeding. Typically you will be put on blood thinners either the day of or the day after joint replacement surgery to help prevent DVT or PE. The type of blood thinner and duration of blood thinner treatment will depend on your individual risk factors and surgeon's preference. There are other techniques beyond the scope of this handbook that we may employ to help, and there are whole families of new drugs being developed which will mitigate these issues even more.

Infection

Infection is a risk when you have surgery. Infection occurs about 1 percent of the time after knee replacement, and is slightly less common after hip replacement. It's not that we don't try to prevent infection—we do. In my practice we do a number of things to help mitigate the risk. Patients are screened for *methicillin resistant staphylococcus aureus* (MRSA) upon arrival to the hospital (MRSA is a drug resistant type of bacteria responsible for wound infections). On the day of surgery, all of my patients have IV antibiotics administered before the operation begins so the antibiotics are in the blood stream before the time of the incision. These antibiotics are usually continued for twenty-four hours after surgery. My entire surgical team and I wear "space suits," which are enclosed helmets and gowns that do not allow (for example) even so much as a flake of dandruff to fall into the wound and cause infection. We clip the hair on the hip or knee and prepare the skin with a sterilizing agent. We even use rooms with special air-flow patterns called "laminar flow rooms" to help reduce the amount of bacteria suspended in the air at any given time in the OR. I also put antibiotics in the cement we use to adhere the joint replacement parts to the bone. This is only a small portion of our efforts to reduce risk for infection. A lot of what we do is beyond the scope of this book. Suffice it to say that we surgeons hate infection and do everything we can to prevent it.

How do you know you have an infection? Well, sometimes it's obvious and sometimes it's not. In general the signs of infection are fever (usually above 101°F), increasing pain (you will have pain, but is the pain worsening?), increasing drainage (again, a small amount of drainage is normal for the first few days after surgery, but it should not be worsening), and increased redness. If you suspect or fear that you may have an infection, contact your doctor's office for an evaluation. It is advantageous to catch infections early, as the treatment is easier if caught sooner. Once an infection has settled deep into the joint replacement this sometimes necessitates removal of the joint replacement to cure the infection. The reason that infection can be such a problem in joint replacements is that infection can "stick" to metal. Some infections can even form protective layers over themselves, allowing them to resist the effects of antibiotics.

Holland's Comment: It's possible that your surgeon will require examination by your dentist to determine the health of your teeth and gums before surgery. It's important to tell your surgeon if you have any active dental infections. If your mouth, gums, and teeth aren't healthy, they are a portal for infection. After your TKR or THR your surgeon may also require you to take antibiotics prior to having any dental work done to prevent infection. Dr. Hugate covers this more in *Chapter 16, Life After Joint Replacement.*

Another issue emerging over the last couple of decades is that of antibiotic resistant bacteria. MRSA (Methicillin Resistant Staphyloccus Aureus) is one such example. This is a common bacterium (staph) that has evolved to be resistant to some antibiotics. Here is an analogy that may help you understand how this occurs: Suppose you owned an island, and on that island were thousands of beautiful red and yellow tulips. What would happen if you sprayed the island with a plant spray that was toxic to the red tulips? Well, the red tulips would all disappear. Over time, the island would repopulate with only—you got it—yellow tulips. The yellow tulips would all be *resistant* to the plant spray. One way of describing this scenario is to say that the yellow tulips were *selected* for survival by the plant spray.

Now let's apply that same logic to bacteria. If a bacteria is treated with an antibiotic that kills most (but not all) of the bacteria, only those bacteria able to resist the antibiotic will survive. You are then left with a few resistant bacteria. They will divide, however, over time and their offspring will possess those same resistance characteristics. Pretty soon you have a full-blown infection with resistant bacteria! Again, the bacteria were selected for survival by the antibiotic. Because modern medical antibiotics have been around for almost ninety years, we are starting to see resistant strains of common bacteria emerge. The pharmaceutical industry fights this by constantly developing new drugs—a new mousetrap, so to speak. So fortunately, we usually have a drug or drugs that can treat most infections, but it is an issue to be aware of.

Joint Stiffness

Joint stiffness is a risk mainly after knee replacement. This is not a common issue after hip replacement. What I mean by "stiffness" is that you do not regain adequate knee motion after surgery. This can be due to a number of factors. One factor that contributes heavily to this (that you cannot change) is that of genetics. Some people are genetically programmed to make thick, dense scar tissue after injuries or surgery. If this is the case with you, you must be doubly vigilant about adhering to a strict and aggressive physical therapy regimen. You should also consider what your knee range of motion was before surgery. If you came into knee replacement with only 90 degrees of motion, you will have a harder time getting the typical 130 degrees of motion after surgery. There are technical reasons for stiffness as well. Knee replacement parts that are too big can also cause stiffness.

Another common cause of stiffness is non-compliance—when a patient does not follow the postoperative physical therapy orders. The bottom line is:

If you don't follow the advice of your treatment team regarding physical therapy and home exercises, you may be disappointed in your range of motion.

I always tell my patients to focus on the straightening of the knee. It is harder to get your knee fully straight after surgery than it is to get it fully bent, and not being able to fully straighten your knee can be miserable. It causes pain and fatigue in your leg that can limit your ability to walk distances. And it's not easy to correct. You will have about an eight-week window after surgery in which you can work to get your knee motion back. Any motion you do not have by then, you will likely not get unless you have another surgery. That's why it's imperative to dedicate yourself to that goal for the first two months after your knee replacement.

Hip Dislocation

Dislocation of the joint is a risk after hip replacement surgery. As described previously, the hip is a ball and socket joint. A dislocation of the hip is when the ball comes out of the socket, and it is usually felt immediately by the patient as severe hip pain. The leg will also shorten (by an inch or two) right away if this happens. This occurs less than 1 percent of the time after hip replacement surgery. There are a number of reasons why a patient may dislocate his hip, but by far the most common reason is called "postural indiscretion." This means that the patient put his hip in an "unstable position" which caused it to pop out of joint. We describe the unstable positions and the *Hip Precautions* in *Chapter 14, Physical Therapy for Hip and Knee Replacement Surgery*. Other causes of dislocation include trauma, poor positioning of the hip replacement components, infection, nerve damage, or muscle damage. In general, hip dislocation occurs more frequently right after surgery and less frequently the further you get out from surgery. The risk for dislocation never goes to zero, though, so people with hip replacements must be careful to observe the **Hip Precautions** for the rest of their lives.

Leg Length Differences

Another risk more specific to hip replacement patients is that of leg length inequality. Before I comment further let me say that, in normal humans, leg lengths on the same person often vary by one-quarter to one-half inch naturally—meaning that one leg is usually somewhat longer than the other. When the hip is replaced, we surgeons have many decisions to make. What size cup, what size ball, the stem, and so on. These can all affect the overall length of your leg. When we select the components, our first priority is to make the hip stable (less likely to dislocate). Our second priority is to ensure that the leg length is correct. Most often we are able to achieve both, but on occasion a hip must be made longer in order to make it more stable. If the leg lengths are off by more than a half an inch, you may notice it. You will feel "lopsided" when you walk, or even have to swing the leg out abnormally to take steps. If this occurs the remedy is to put a thin heel cushion in the shoe of your shorter leg. This will effectively equalize the leg lengths and make your gait feel more normal. On rare occasion, if the difference is bigger, the surgeon will have to go back in with surgery and change some of the components to shorten the leg. This occurs less than 1 percent of the time in hip replacement surgery.

Nerve and Blood Vessel Issues

Any time you have surgery there is a risk of damaging major nerves or blood vessels. This is exceedingly rare during hip and knee replacements, but the risk is not zero. The risk of having major damage to the nerves or blood vessels during a hip or knee replacement is less than 0.5 percent. The major nerves and blood vessels in the leg are situated behind the knee and are therefore relatively well protected during TKR. However, there are major nerves both in front of and behind your hip. If major blood vessels were injured during surgery, another surgeon, known as a vascular surgeon, may be able to repair the vessel, but it would not be without additional incisions and a lengthier and potentially more complicated recovery process.

If nerves were to become damaged, this would cause numbness or weakness of the leg and foot below the level of the injury. The symptoms of nerve injury are reversible if the nerve is only bruised, but the nerve symptoms can be permanent if the nerve is completely cut. One thing you will almost certainly see in a *normal,* uncomplicated

227

joint replacement is some numbness around the incision. This is more common in knee replacement surgery than hip replacement surgery, but it can be experienced in both. In the knee, there is often a patch of numbness along the outside of the knee. This is because the skin incision required to perform a joint replacement cuts across some small hair-like nerves in the skin. Again, if you experience this, it is normal. The numbness improves over time, but usually never returns completely to normal.

Implant Failure or Loosening

An exceedingly rare risk of hip and knee replacement surgery is that of implant failure. Joint replacements are made of metal, plastic, and sometimes even ceramics. These materials are capable of bending, fatiguing, cracking and/or failing—just like any part in your car. They are built to high tolerance and have safety mechanisms built into them through their engineering but still, a very small percent of these parts can fail. As time goes on, the implant companies get feedback from patients with their implants and make the necessary changes to accommodate for any weakness. On rare occasion an implant will actually be recalled for a number of reasons. Your surgeon and hospital keep records of which implants were used in your joint replacement and should notify you if any of these parts have been recalled. But if you hear about a recall and want to verify, I encourage you to contact your surgeon's office. Again, this is a rare event but should be considered.

In the long term, loosening of the implant is a risk. Joint replacements are either cemented to the bone using a substance called *methyl methacrylate*, or simply "press fit" into place (where the implant *locks* into the bone surface by friction and the bone then grows into it). In either event, the success of the joint replacement is tied to how well the parts adhere to the bone. If a part loosens, it can cause pain. The reasons for loosening are varied and include infection, obesity, plastic wear (the plastic particles generated when the plastic spacer is worn can cause loosening), impact activities (such as running), misalignment of the implants, metal allergy, and traumatic injury.

After your joint is replaced, you will be seen on a regular basis by your surgeon for rechecks. During that visit you will get an X-ray that allows your doctor to check for loosening. Of course, if you have new pains in the hip or knee before your annual checkup, you should make a special appointment to have the joint replacement examined. The solution to a loosened implant depends on a number of factors such as magnitude of pain, the amount of loosening, and the presence of infection. This is the most common long-term complication of knee replacement. The chance your joint replacement will need to be revised due to late loosening is in the range of 2 percent.

Bone Fracture (breaking)

Fracturing (or breaking the bone) during the operation is also a small risk, with an incidence of about 2-3 percent. It is more commonly seen in hip replacements and usually occurs while impacting the parts into place: the bone can simply crack. This may occur for a number of reasons. The bone may be of poor quality (osteoporotic), or the surgeon may simply hit the implant into position too hard. Again, this is rare. The solution is to fix the broken bone during the same operation with plates, screws, or cables. The way the bone is repaired depends on the size, shape, and location of the break. If this occurs, your surgeon will discuss it with you after surgery, describe what problem occurred, and go over the implications with you. Most often, it will require that you limit your weight-bearing on that particular joint until the broken bone has healed, in most cases around six weeks.

Revision Joint Replacement

Let's talk briefly now about "revision" joint replacement. Simply put, this is a surgical procedure in which some or all of the original joint replacement implant is removed and swapped out for new parts. Revision joint surgery may be necessary after joint replacements for a number of reasons. For example, if the plastic spacer in your knee replacement or the plastic cup in your hip replacement is worn down, you can have those parts swapped out for new ones. Similarly, if parts of the joint replacement loosen, are too big or too small, or if they were misaligned, they too can be swapped out. Revision joint replacement is also sometimes necessary in the case of deep joint replacement infections where the implant components have to be removed to allow the infection to clear. Because this is a re-operation, the surgery generally takes longer, the complication rate is a bit higher, and the recovery is slower than a first-time joint replacement surgery.

Loss of Limb

A few of my patients ask me, "Doc, is there any chance that I could lose my leg if I have a joint replacement?" This is an important question, and the answer is yes, it is *possible*— but again, exceedingly rare. This is a worse-case scenario that can become reality, but only if a number of things go wrong at once. For example, if your knee becomes infected and that infection persists despite multiple attempts at eradicating it, then amputation may be necessary. Also, if you suffered any severe damage to your nerves or blood vessels that (for whatever reason) turned out to be irreparable, this could lead to amputation. But all of these situations are highly unlikely to occur.

Summary

To summarize, these are the main surgical risks to be aware of if you choose to undergo joint replacement surgery. Remember, about 95 percent of patients undergoing joint replacement surgery enjoy good to excellent results with no major complications, so keep it all in perspective.

> **We continue to make strides in all fields of medicine and surgery to help reduce all potential risks.**

Lastly, the potential for issues I have covered in this chapter are for the general population. If you have any unusual medical conditions, this may increase (or decrease) your risk for any particular complication. It's extremely important that you discuss your individual situation with your surgeon and his treatment team prior to considering surgery. Please consider these possibilities when making your decision as to whether to proceed with joint replacement surgery.

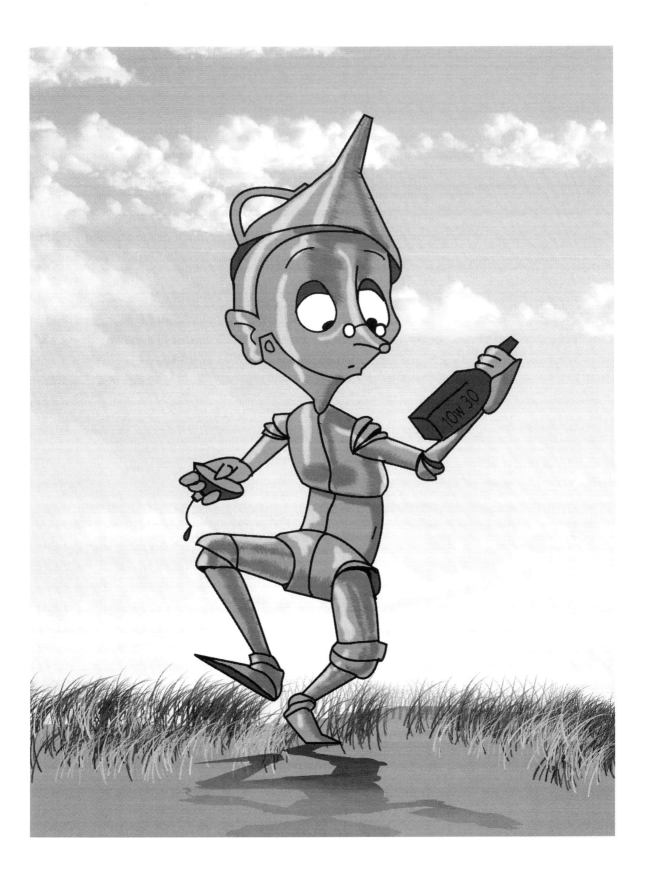

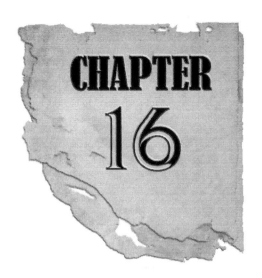

Life After Joint Replacement

by Dr. Hugate

CHAPTER 16

Whew, you've made it! All of the time you spent preparing, rehabilitating, and healing was worth it. The joint replacement is behind you and you can now go on living your life without the pain. Enjoy it, you deserve it! And that's the whole reason you put yourself through surgery. Now you can be yourself again.

Even though you're done with your joint replacement, there are some things you need to be aware of going forward. Not too much to know—just a few minor issues. This chapter of the handbook will address the ongoing maintenance of your joint replacement after you've fully recovered from THR or TKR and also identify a few "land mines" for you to dodge. Keeping a copy of this handbook and looking back on this chapter every so often is not a bad idea. Having a knee or hip replacement is like buying a new car in many ways. I'll use this analogy to help you understand the "upkeep" necessary from here on out.

First of all, when should you see your surgeon? Like the parts of a car, the parts of your knee replacement can wear out over time. It's much easier to address this problem if it's discovered early. The typical knee or hip replacement these days lasts about fifteen years on average. Once a joint replacement is worn out, it may need to have some "maintenance" done on it. This is rare, but again, if worn parts are caught early it's much easier for both the patient and the surgeon to fix things before they get worse. For these reasons, joint replacement surgeons these days typically see their patients back routinely once a year or once every two years for follow up. Now, if you have an appointment with your orthopedic surgeon but something new comes up in the meantime (such as pain, stiffness, swelling, or instability), then you should call his office or simply go back to see him sooner.

Now, let's talk about your dental health. I can hear your thoughts: "Dental health? What does my dental health have to do with my joint replacement?" If it's bad, it can have a lot to do with your joint replacement. You see, one of the ongoing risks after having a joint replacement is that it could still become infected. How? Well, here is an example of how it usually happens: A hip replacement patient may go to her dentist for a professional cleaning or a more major dental procedure. During the procedure the gums bleed. This allows access for bacteria in your mouth to get into your bloodstream. It's like opening a door for an army of bacteria to walk through and get into your bloodstream. Remember from **Chapter 15, What Can Go Wrong?** that bacteria *love* metal. They can travel through your bloodstream and land on that metal implant and literally *stick* to it. This could cause a deep infection of your joint replacement that's very difficult to fight.

How can you avoid this trouble? First, see your dentist regularly to ensure that you have no active infections in your mouth and keep your teeth clean.

Holland's Comment: You must take Dr. Hugate's advice about dental hygiene very seriously. Personally, I use a water-jet, flossing appliance, every morning (there are several brands available) and I use a light solution of of my favorite mouthwash in it. The water-jet pumping action cleans around the periphery of the transition between teeth and gums. Use a light setting so as not to damage the gums at first. These days I use it on the highest setting. This would be a good habit to start before your TKR or THR and continue forever. ~*~

If you have any dental procedures performed (including professional cleaning) make sure your dentist knows you have a joint replacement. You should receive antibiotics before having the procedure done. They can be prescribed either by your dentist or your orthopedic surgeon's office. The goal is to have the antibiotic in your blood stream *before* the procedure so that any bacteria getting into your bloodstream *during* the procedure will be killed by the antibiotic before they get to your joint replacement. For my patients, I recommend that they get antibiotics prior to any dental procedures for the rest of their lives. Some orthopedic surgeons recommend antibiotics only for a prescribed amount of time after your joint replacement is done. Please check with your surgeon and ask for how long before minor procedures he would like you to take antibiotics.

The same argument holds true for any invasive medical procedure, not just for dental procedures. Any procedure that will potentially break the skin and allow bacteria to enter the blood stream should be treated the same way. Examples are colonoscopy, biopsy, mole removal, cystoscopy, hemorrhoid surgery, and eye surgery. If you're unsure if you need antibiotics, call your surgeon's office and discuss it with your treatment team.

234

OK, so what can you do now that your joint is replaced? Remember the goal of the operation was to improve your pain and deformity, *not* to make you a professional athlete. Your hip or knee will feel better than it has in years. For some, that equals a license to get rowdy. Don't get me wrong, you went through this so that you could be active, and I want you to be active—but there's a *limit* to what you should be doing. I generally draw the line at impact activities. This includes running, jumping, jogging, and any sport which requires an abrupt twist, turn, or stop. Skiing is OK as long as you're reasonable and avoid the jumps, moguls, and black/blue slopes.

Why do we limit you? Impact activities can wear your joint replacement out far too soon. Remember the car analogy from *Chapter 12, Methods, Types and Designs of Joint Replacements*? You just got a new car and the tires are brand new. You can wear those tires out in a short time or they can last you for years. It depends on how aggressively you drive, right? If you drive only on paved roads and obey the speed limit, your tires will last a long time. If you go off road and/or race the car, the tires won't last long and will need early replacement. Get it? The same is true for the parts of your joint replacement. Treat your joint well, and you could get fifteen or more years out of it. Treat it poorly and I'll be seeing you back sooner for re-treading.

For those of you who've had your hips replaced: please continue to follow your hip precautions. Remember, the hip precautions are a series of positions to avoid after having a hip replacement. These are described well in *Chapter 14, Physical Therapy for Hip and Knee Replacement* of this handbook. If you put your hip in one of these positions, it could dislocate—even many years after surgery. The risk of dislocating your hip does go down significantly after the first three months following surgery, but the risk never goes to zero. If you dislocate your hip, correcting the problem requires, at the very least, that you be sedated to put the hip back in the joint and sometimes even requires surgery to put it back. Learn and live the hip precautions taught to you by your physical therapist. For most patients, they become second nature after a few weeks, and the patients never even have to think about them anymore.

Another issue that comes up commonly in follow-up is that of noise. Joint replacements tend to make a lot of funny noises. Pops, clicks, and thumps are all par for the course. Remember that the joint replacement is made of metal, plastic, and sometimes ceramic. When these substances come into contact you may feel and hear a click. This is generally nothing to be alarmed about unless it's painful. There is also a phenomenon known as the "squeaking hip." This was initially described in the 1990s and is almost exclusively seen with ceramic on ceramic hip replacements. These were hip replacements in which the ball and the socket were both replaced with ceramic parts. Again, this isn't a dangerous phenomenon, but the sound is irritating. I encourage you to discuss any sounds you hear with your doctor, but take some comfort in the fact that these implants tend to make noise and unless it is painful it's usually normal and does not require any intervention.

Some patients ask me what can be done about their scar in the long term. The answer is really not much. Your scar is more a result of your genetics than anything else. I suture my patients' incisions the same way every time. Some people heal up and you can barely see their scar. Others have a thick scar that persists. I know it may seem as though I am passing blame on here, but I'm simply stating fact. The scar will continue to evolve and change for about a full year after surgery. The scar tends to be thickest in the first three months and then "mature" and flatten over time. Initially the scars have a reddish or purple appearance and that too fades over the first year. When you get to the one-year anniversary, your scar is about as good as it's going to get. In the meantime, scar massage and even application of vitamin E or aloe based lotions seem to help a bit. Don't start putting lotions or creams on your wound until you get the OK from your surgeon. One way to predict what your scar may look like after surgery is to look at your previous scars, either from previous surgery or after a deep cut that you suffered in the past.

You should also continue your routine health maintenance under your PCP's care. Now that your hip or knee feels better, try to get out and walk often. This will help you reduce your weight and (along with a number of other benefits) will allow your joint replacement to last longer. If you are a diabetic, keep your blood sugars under control. Also diabetics and people with poor circulation should watch their feet very carefully. Ulcers can occur on the legs and feet of people with diabetes or vascular problems because the blood flow is limited and some don't have normal sensation. Make it a routine to visually inspect your feet daily (or have your significant other do so). Having a skin ulcer of any kind puts your joint replacement at high risk for infection. If you notice an ulcer or skin breakdown, see your doctor immediately. Also your PCP will keep you up to date with immunizations to include annual flu vaccines and pneumonia vaccine if appropriate.

Campone's Comment: One more observation which applies to hips and knee replacements: I found that my new bionic body sets off airport scanner alarms every time I travel. While the surgeon did provide a note confirming that I had two THRs, I'm regularly checked by a female Transportation Security Administration agent. So when traveling by airplane, you might want to be prepared and allow a little extra time for the process of having your total joint implants verified. ~*~

Now, take a deep breath, and enjoy your new joint replacement. This can be a new lease on life for many folks. Spend time walking with your loved ones, or playing with your grandchildren. Go on vacation! Go dancing! The worst thing you can do to yourself is go through this arduous process and then not use your new joint.

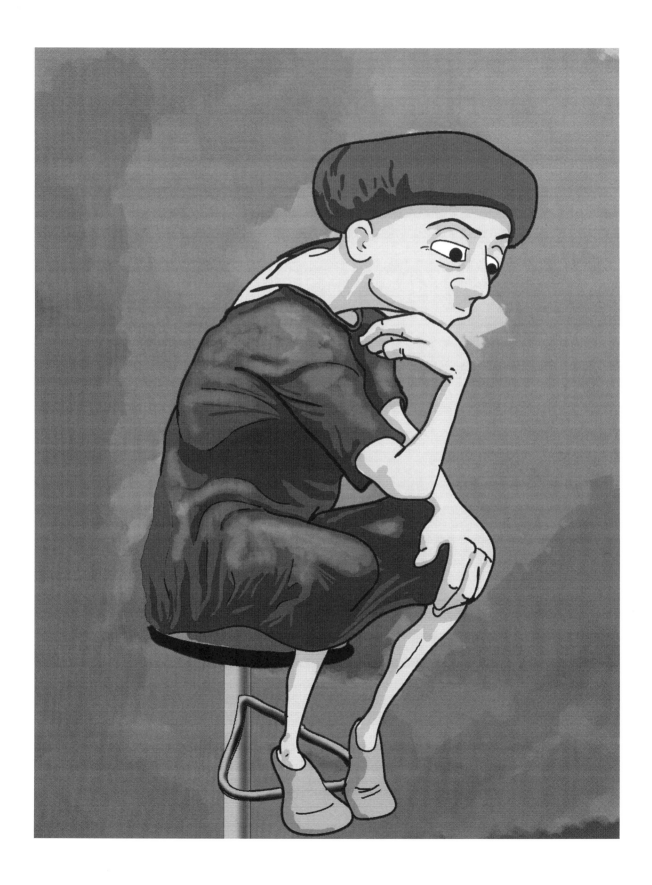

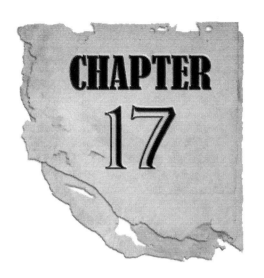

Final Thoughts

by Dr. Hugate and Mr. Holland

Well, that's it, a description of the joint replacement journey from beginning to end. Joint replacement surgery is about the patient and I think it's appropriate to end our handbook with Robert's well-chosen words and perspective. Robert and I have spent countless hours on compiling and presenting this information to you in an understandable and meaningful way. I truly believe that if you've read this handbook, you'll be as prepared as you can be heading into the journey through joint replacement.

Use the information as a springboard for discussion with your surgeon about your personal situation. Every patient is different and has unique issues and concerns. This handbook is not an exhaustive source of information about the intricacies of joint replacement, but rather written to familiarize you with the majority of the facts and facets and get you in the game.

My father used to tell me, "Nothing worth doing is ever easy." Joint replacement is certainly no exception. Although techniques in surgery and pain management have advanced a great deal in recent years, it's still surgery and—as always—there are risks associated with any course of treatment. But with the information presented in this handbook you can make a knowledgeable and well-considered decision. For patients with painful, debilitating arthritis of the hip or knee, joint replacement surgery can open up a whole new world. Use your newfound understanding to help guide and inform you through the decision-making process. I wish you all the best in your personal quest for improved quality of life and pain relief.

Today Vicki and I, and my Labs went for a hike in the high, Colorado woods. The altitude was around 8,500 feet and it was a blustery day around noon—almost cold—yet there was a tinge of the warmth to come in the approaching spring air. When I hike here in the wonderful parks and woods around Denver, I never give a thought to the fact that my knee has been replaced. Forgetting completely about it, I look around me at the amazing Rocky Mountain scenery and listen to the pines whispering loudly in the stiff breeze. I ponder how much joy I get from just watching my brown Lab, Casey, romping, jumping, and basically running amuck in the open space around us. Our older Black Lab, Roxy, sticks close by as we hike straight up the steep dirt road to the top of our mountain objective. We can see all the way to Denver from here—many, many miles! The trail then takes us back down the other side of the peak and slowly curves back around after about a mile. We end up near a small, babbling, mountain brook, just now beginning to trickle and flow again after the winter stilled it as a frozen piece of white, crystalline, winter's art. Today I contemplated how it had stopped flowing for a time, like my own life had done, and how it was coming back to itself as the small and quiet beginning of some larger river far away downstream.

We stopped at the bottom of the trail and stood there a while, as we always do, while the dogs ran about sniffing this, investigating that, and I realized what a wonderful gift I've been given. Were it not for my joint replacement, I wouldn't be able to enjoy this wondrous and beautiful place anymore. I'd miss the peppery, alpine smell of the deep, coniferous woods, the enchanting color of the light green rock-moss glistening with dew drops in the sun, and the delicious warmth of the spring sun on my face. I had lost the ability to hike to this place years before we wrote this handbook, when my knee was so painful I couldn't do any of the outdoor activities I so love. I couldn't even walk at the mall or do a complete workout at our local wellness center. This, then, was a time for reflection, gratitude, grace, and contemplation on what I've been newly given and what I once gave up.

I remembered how I asked myself whether I felt—in my heart—strong enough to make that journey in regaining these things I love so much. My new knee isn't perfectly pain free; sometimes it aches a bit, and sometimes it gets cold in the frosty depths of the Colorado winter, and sometimes in the shimmering heat of summer it gets too hot. But when I climb the big stairs at the movie theater, or at Coors Field for a Colorado Rockies baseball game, and I climb them just as easily and quickly as everybody else, without ever a thought about the journey behind me, I find myself in the perfect moment—just being there, being me. As we age, I believe we begin to see time differently—we develop perspective. Here then, is my advice. Remember in my introduction where I made the metaphor about life being a voyage on a river. I'll expand on that now that you've pretty much finished our handbook.

If life is a river and you're on a raft floating along, the river of life always has a flow—whether you can sense it or not. It has hidden currents and unknown dangers.

You've never been down this river before and you don't know where it comes out, what's in store, or what adventures or challenges it'll bring along the way. Sometimes a fork you've chosen turns out to be a dead-end backwater and you have to paddle your way back out. Sometimes you go over the falls kicking and screaming, or down the rapids whooping and hollering, but the changes that occur cannot be undone—there's no going back. The past can't be undone, leaving you only and always in the present, flowing right along with the current and only ever able to affect the future course of your existence on this river of life. What you *do* know is that many challenges will surely be ahead and undertaking a joint replacement is simply one more of the many profound challenges in your life. This river of life has forks, and the fork you choose, while looking ahead and planning your course, makes all the difference. You won't know if you've chosen the serene lake or the roaring rapids until you go around the bend—that's the adventure and excitement of it all.

For those on this float trip with you, remember that what happens to you happens to them—you're in the boat together. While many others tie up alongside for a time, they'll eventually go their own way, but your *loved ones* are there until the float trip is over.

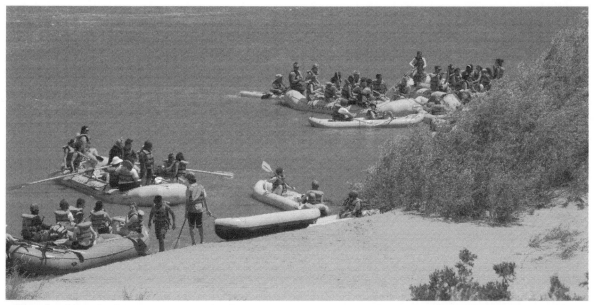

On the beach for some rest before traveling on, Colorado River in Castle Valley, Utah.

Of course, sometimes the waters are calm, peaceful, and clear, but sometimes chaotic, fierce, and dark. These are the times when you must plan and work together in harmony with both the people in your boat and those tied up alongside. Remember to include and empower them all to help you navigate and set your course, but listen to your own voice too. After all, you're the captain. When you do these things, you'll achieve some wisdom in finding the right branch of the river. Your objective—whether you choose joint replacement or not—is to find someplace where you can once again experience your own "peak moments."

We've been very thorough in preparing you for this float trip. We've told you how to plan your quest and empowered you in making it to your destination. This is because, like all good river guides, we've been down this branch of the river before. Our combined wisdom, thoughts, experiences, and knowledge have led you to this moment, and it's time to ask yourself the following questions.

Why am I here?

What's brought me to this place in my life's journey?

What's my purpose in embarking on this new journey through total joint replacement?

How will my life change if I do?

What will happen if I don't?

How you answer these compelling questions will determine what branch of the river of life you take next, so remember to be looking forward, in the direction of the flow, not backward wishing in vain you could have changed your course—this river only flows in one direction… into the future. Keep on commanding your own course—you're doing fine as the captain of your life—who could do better? One last thought, *nobody ever said it was going to be easy*. You'll always challenge yourself by making the choices that create new adventures like this.

Oh, and be sure to splash someone you love every once in a while just for fun.

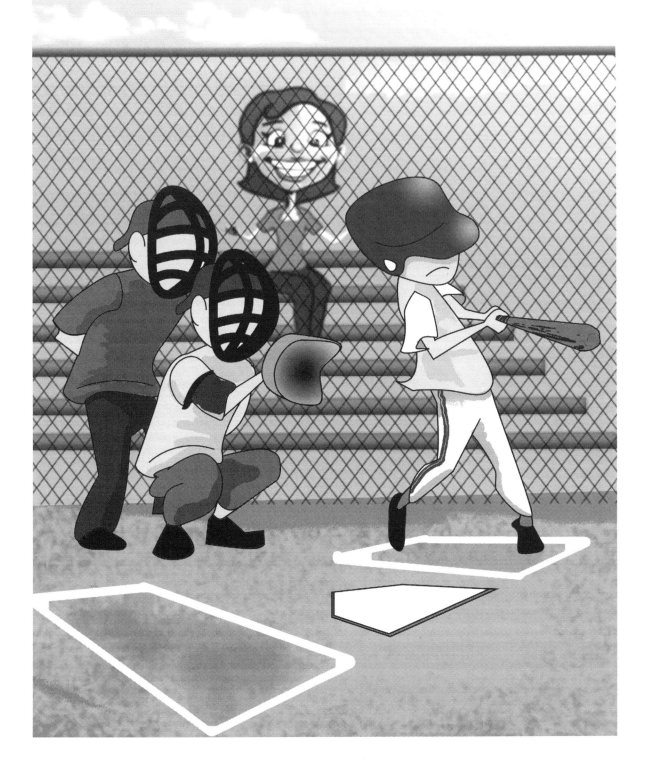

Getting to Know Our Team

CHAPTER 18

Ronald R. Hugate Jr., MD

Dr. Hugate is the Chairman of Orthopedic Surgery at Presbyterian/Saint Luke's Medical Center in Denver, Colorado. Following residency in orthopedic surgery at Penn State, he completed a two-year fellowship at the Mayo Clinic in 2005. He then moved to Denver to join Colorado Limb Consultants and is a member physician of the Denver Clinic for Extremities at Risk. He specializes in joint replacements, complex orthopedic problems, and treatment of tumors involving the muscles and joints.

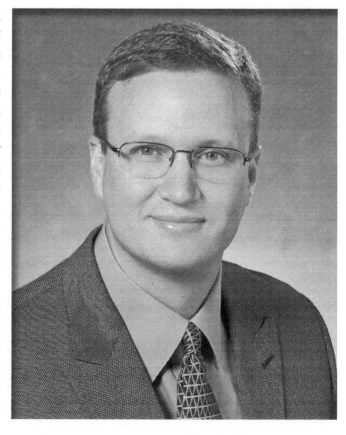

His research interests involve advancement of joint replacement design technology and the treatment of bone cancers. He has published numerous scientific articles and spoken on various subjects at academic conferences.

Dr. Hugate was born in Virginia and is married with three children. He enjoys spending time with his family, classic American muscle cars, scuba diving, wood-working, and skiing. He is also a Lieutenant Colonel in the U.S. Army Reserves and has served in Iraq and Afghanistan at combat surgical hospitals supporting our troops. He has been awarded numerous honors, including two Army Commendation medals for his meritorious service.

Robert Holland, PMP

Robert attended the University of Colorado and graduated Magna Cum Laude with a Bachelor of Science in Information Systems. In this capacity, he performed information technology (IT) consulting and owned an IT consulting company until early 2002, when he settled down for a long and fruitful employment with the State of Colorado sheriffs association where he was the Director of Information Services and

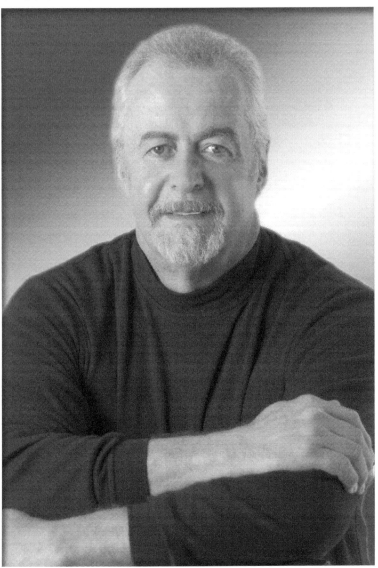

the IT Project Manager. He eventually earned his Project Management Professional (PMP) Certification in mid-2009.

Robert has been both a writer of science fiction (as a hobby) and a technical writer (as part of his information systems career). Robert is an avid bicyclist (on the many bike trails around his home in Denver Colorado) and loves to hike in the beautiful and rugged Colorado Rockies. Robert's favorite vacation is to take Vicki and their two Labrador Retrievers and travel up the Pacific Coast Highway from northern California through Oregon and Washington states with their twenty-four-foot travel trailer. He also loves the Canyonlands National Park near Moab, Utah, where he and Vicki both enjoy the rewarding hobby of digital photography—and more hiking.

Francine Campone, EdD

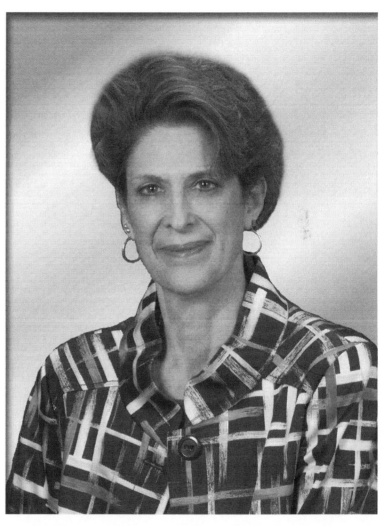

Francine Campone, EdD, provides executive and personal coaching to mature professionals making career and life transitions. She is no stranger to transitions, moving from her hometown of Brooklyn, New York, to Rapid City, South Dakota, where she lived for fifteen years before moving with her husband to Denver, Colorado. Francine's professional journey includes a thirty-plus-year career in higher and adult education and formal coach training, complemented by training in humanistic mediation, group dynamics and facilitation, and Constructive Living Practice. Francine believes that change can not only be managed but can be turned into opportunities that might have otherwise been missed. In 2001, she started her own small coaching and consulting company and enjoys her work with clients in the corporate, nonprofit, and education sectors across the United States. Her total hip replacement experience offered an opportunity to upgrade her physical self-care, lose weight, and start a daily morning stretching routine. Francine is also a creative knitter and is on the journey of learning how to weave.

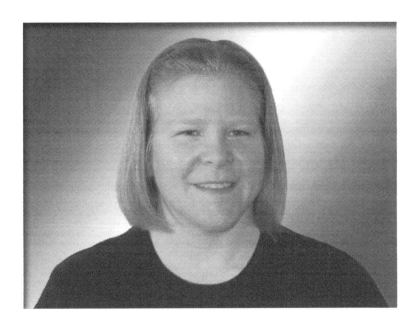

Inger Brueckner, MSPT

Inger grew up in a small town in northern California and graduated from the University of California at Davis (UC Davis) with a Bachelor of Science in Physiology. While at UC Davis, she also played saxophone in the California Aggie Marching Band. She then traveled to the East Coast and graduated from Boston University with a Master of Science in Physical Therapy. After her time in Boston, MA, she moved to San Diego, CA, and lived by the beach for almost two years. Inger grew up near Dodge Ridge Ski Resort and Yosemite National Park, and while living by the beach she eventually began to miss the mountains, so she moved to Denver in 1994. She now enjoys the Colorado outdoors experience with her husband and son whenever they can get away. Inger has worked as a physical therapist in many different kinds of settings and always enjoys new challenges. She currently works at Presbyterian/St. Luke's (P/SL) Medical Center at the Rehabilitation & Sports Medicine Center and has been at P/SL since 2005. She often takes continuing education classes in order to advance her treatment techniques, knowledge, skills, and abilities, and has lectured nationally on vestibular rehabilitation and amputee rehabilitation. For the past eighteen years, she has seen total joint replacement patients in a variety of settings, including inpatient hospital, rehabilitation hospitals, home health settings and outpatient clinics.

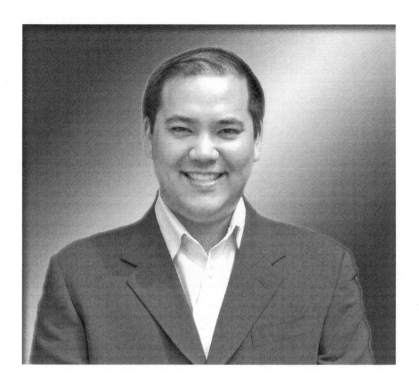

Giancarlo Checa, MD

Dr. Checa is an anesthesiologist with a subspecialty in pain management. He practices in Denver and is a member of Metro Denver Anesthesia. He was raised in southern California and attended medical school at the University of Colorado Health Sciences Center. He then completed an Anesthesia Residency at Yale. Afterward, he completed a Pain Management Fellowship at University of California San Francisco. Dr. Checa provides anesthesia for in-patient and outpatient surgeries. He also has a pain management practice with Metro Denver Pain.

Dr. Checa was born in Panama and speaks Spanish. He is married with two children. He enjoys spending time with his family, hiking, skiing, and traveling.

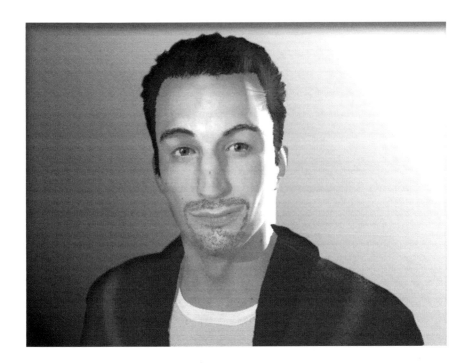

Ryan Counts, CGA

Ryan graduated from high school in Denver, Colorado and completed an Associate Degree in Applied Science from Wyotech technical institute in Laramie, Wyoming. In 2005, Ryan moved to Phoenix, Arizona where he then earned a Bachelor of Arts in Media Art & Animation. This is where he and some fellow class mates started Endemic Studios, a commercial studio focusing on animations and visual aids for small business advertising. This gave Ryan the opportunity to work on story boarding, character animation, character design, and 3D modeling.

Ryan now lives in Denver, Colorado, working as a freelance, computer graphics artist. It was here that he began working with this handbook's coauthor, Robert Holland, creating covers for Robert's science fiction novels. It was through his work with Robert that Ryan was invited to illustrate this handbook.

Ryan has greatly enjoyed illustrating this handbook drawing on both his talent for technical illustration and his great sense of humor for cartooning—all to bring these complex issues to life and help lighten the tone of the subject matter as well. He is honored to use his artistic abilities for the many folks out there using this handbook to guide them through a real life journey.

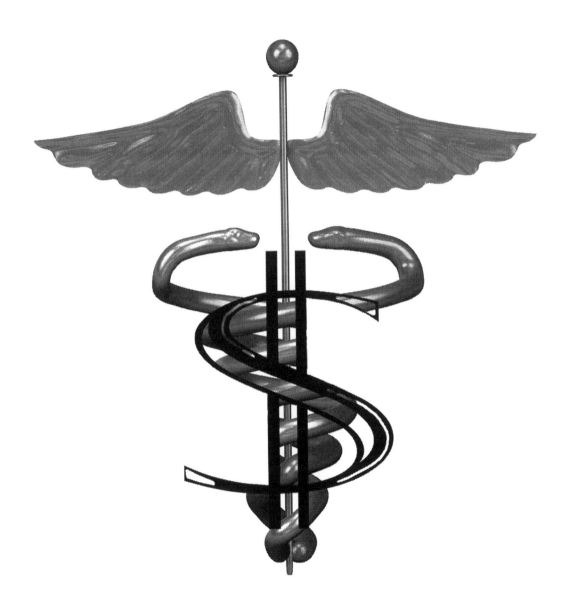

INSURANCE

Insurance Matters

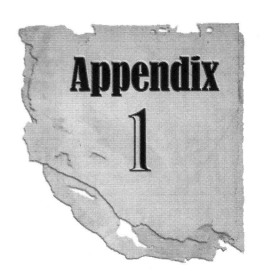

Appendix 1

by Dr. Hugate

H ealth care insurance is getting a lot of attention these days. Believe me, this is not one of my favorite topics, but it's a *practical* topic that must be considered before committing to joint replacement surgery. This is also *not* a topic to ignore and hope for the best. The high costs of medical care can get out of hand very quickly. If you don't carefully scrutinize your coverage and have everything pre-approved, you may be stuck holding a very big bag. What I will try to do here is very briefly introduce you to common medical coverage issues we see with our patients in the clinic. Again, since my practice is in the USA, much of what we discuss here will be more applicable to Americans.

Preparing For the Operation

When preparing for surgery, it's important for you to know some basic information about your health insurance coverage and benefit information. First of all, most insurance plans carry a calendar year deductible. A deductible is the amount of money you must pay (out-of-pocket) before the insurance company starts paying their share. The deductible is usually an annual total that accumulates over the calendar year. For example, if your deductible for visits to your PCP is $500, and you visited your PCP once in March and once in July at $150 per visit, you have met $300 of your annual deductible. You still have another $200 to spend out-of-pocket before your insurance starts picking up their share of the tab. Your out-of-pocket deductible resets to the original amount on January 1st with most insurance plans.

253

Know Your Deductibles

Knowing your deductibles, the components and limitations of your plan is very important for a number of reasons. First, there's a trend toward so-called high deductible health plans. These are insurance plans that have a lower premium (which is what makes them attractive), but make you fork out more in deductibles over the year. So-called health savings plans usually have high deductibles as well. Both types of insurance may influence the timing of your surgery as well. I get more requests for knee and hip joint surgery toward the end of the year because many patients have met their deductibles by then, meaning the surgery will involve less out-of-pocket costs for them. For these types of plans, be sure you know what your deductible is, and how much of it has been satisfied for the year.

Know Your Maximum Yearly Limits

In many cases, modern insurance policies may have a maximum number of visits allowed per year for certain types of medical services (such as twenty visits per year to the physical therapist). Be aware of this, as it may limit your options. For example, if you have two knee replacements in one year, each several months apart, and you're limited to twenty visits per year to the physical therapist (in total), you'll only have ten visits per operation. If everything goes well, this may be adequate. If you need more, it becomes your burden to pay the difference. This can be a reason to plan your surgery in the second half of the year. If you end up needing more visits—say, for the physical therapist—the period of need spans from one year to the next. This is another example of how limitations on specific services might influence the timing of your operation. Your insurance carrier should have all of this information and be willing to help you figure out your options.

Holland's Comment: Something that I've learned the hard way is to keep a "medical journal" every year (think: diary or trip-log with associated costs, like service calls to the shop for your car). I keep track of my doctor's appointments and co-pays and I do this for some very important reasons. First, I can tell where I went, whom I saw, and for what reason. Next, I keep all my co-pays in one spot for tax-time in case we exceed the amount required by the U.S.

Internal Revenue Service for the Standard Deduction and can itemize our combined medical expenses. Assembling all of this can be difficult to collate at tax time once your preparer tells you it's OK. So, if you have your medical journal, finding the supporting bills and insurance summary-sheets is much easier. ~*~

Coinsurance and Copay

Another term that you need to become familiar with is "coinsurance." Most insurance plans require that you personally pay a certain dollar amount each year over and above your deductible. This is called your coinsurance. For example, many insurance policies are arranged such that, once you meet your deductible, they (the insurance company) will pay 80 percent of the remaining costs while you pay 20 percent coinsurance.

"Co-pay" is similar to coinsurance in the previous example. A co-pay is a certain amount of money that you must pay for each visit with a provider. This is exclusive of what the insurance company pays for your visit. This is another important number for you to be aware of. The charges for surgery can mount up, and a high coinsurance and co-pays could stress you financially.

Holland's Comment: Many of the modern health insurance plan types (such as Health Maintenance Organization [aka HMO] or Preferred Provider Network [PPN]) which have co-pays may not have a ceiling on your out-of-pocket expenses, so be sure to check. They are often structured in a way that each occurrence or visit to the doctor's office, hospital, physical therapist, and/or other specialists have a more reasonable, smaller percentage cost per visit. ~*~

The saving grace of co-pay and coinsurance is the so-called maximum out-of-pocket expense. This is a dollar amount, set by your policy carrier, which is the most amount of money you would ever have to pay in a calendar year toward your medical bills. Most insurance will pick up 100 percent of costs after you have met the maximum annual out-of-pocket number—but you should verify this with your insurance company. If this "ceiling" of costs is low, it benefits you. If it's high, you need to know *how high* because there is a good chance you may not get to that ceiling during your joint replacement.

Forms of Insurance

If your health insurance utilizes a PPN (aka Preferred Provider Network)—as with an HMO (Health Maintenance Organization), PPO (Preferred Provider Organization), POS (Point of Service [plan]), EPO (Exclusive Provider Organization), and so on—it's in your best interest to make sure that all of the providers who will be involved with your care (surgeon, surgical assistant(s), facility/hospital, laboratory, radiologist, anesthesiologist, and so on) participate in your health plan as well. By doing so, you'll be able to maximize your insurance benefits and avoid incurring debt from providers who do not participate with your health insurance's network. This will be an important part of the discussion you have with the surgeon's office staff prior to surgery. They can generally let you know which providers may fall outside of the preferred group, and where possible, direct you to providers that are within your network.

Prior Authorization and Pre-approval

Most insurance plans require prior authorization for both outpatient and inpatient hospital admissions. This means someone from the insurance company needs to be made aware of your intent to have surgery and has to approve (in writing) the visit or surgery before they agree to pay any part of your bill. Most insurance plans impose strict penalties to their members for not honoring the prior authorization policy. In some cases, your health insurance plan may impose a one-time penalty of $250 or $500, or they can reduce the percentage of benefit that they would normally pay on your behalf if you don't pre-approve the care.

The pre-approval process can be simple or complex depending on your situation and your insurance carrier. When you visit your doctor, be sure to have a legible insurance card to present to the front office staff. One of the receptionist's duties is to verify your insurance and let you know if the pre-approval criteria for the visit have been met and what deductible or co-pays are required by your insurance company for your visit. Often you will need a referral from your Primary Care Provider to initially visit with the surgeon, and then the surgeon's office helps with preapproval of the surgery itself. The insurance company may ask to look at your medical record to determine if they will pre-approve your surgery. This initial screening of approvals is usually carried out by a registered nurse who is employed by the insurance carrier. On the rare occasion, the surgeon will actually have to get on the phone with one of the health care specialists at the insurance company (usually a doctor-to-doctor phone call to one of the insurance company's physicians) and discuss it with them personally to obtain approval. Fortunately, most doctor's offices are familiar with the process and usually assist you with the pre-approval process.

Joint replacement surgery is usually pretty straightforward in terms of insurance pre-approval. Most health insurance plans take up to three to five days to conduct a formal review and approval. One issue to be aware of is the "pre-existing condition." Insurance companies run a business and, as such, try to minimize the amount of payouts to policy-holders. This is done in an effort to maximize profits and minimize the premiums of its members. I'm not making a political statement or a statement of my opinion, but rather a statement of fact. For that reason, on occasion, they will scrutinize a request for pre-approval very closely. Some insurances exclude "pre-existing" conditions for coverage. That is to say, if there is any medical record in the past indicating that you may have had arthritis prior to signing on with their insurance policy, and it was not disclosed to them on the policy application, they may have the right to deny approval and coverage. The insurance world is changing as I write this and the pre-existing condition may become a thing of the past (depending on which way the political winds blow), but please be aware of this and make sure you don't fall into this trap.

Once a determination has been made, most health insurance plans provide written confirmation of the actual review and approval process. This document will contain an authorization number and will also outline the number of hospital days that have been approved for your hospital stay after surgery. If your hospital stay extends beyond the number of days that had been approved, make sure notification is made to the surgeon's office staff and/or the hospital personnel while you're still hospitalized so this can be addressed immediately. Most hospitals have a case management department that oversees this process. If your insurance carrier doesn't see the need for you to remain in the hospital, you may have to leave sooner than your surgeon would prefer. In general, the insurance companies are fairly reasonable about this, but if they don't approve of the additional day in the hospital, and you decide to stay anyway, you will get the bill.

Durable Medical Equipment

Most health insurance plans have specific benefit provisions for Durable Medical Equipment (DMEs). These are any splints, immobilizers, braces, crutches, walker, cane, etc., that you may need after surgery. Different policies cover varying amounts of durable medical equipment expenses. If you are undergoing joint replacement surgery, it's important to understand your policy in this regard because you will need DMEs. Also, if you're

257

having a knee replacement, look specifically at coverage for the CPM (continuous passive motion) machine. Some patients are required by their surgeons to use these at home for the days immediately after surgery and this may not be covered by your insurance plan.

Limits on Outpatient Services and Therapy

Some insurance companies require that you use certain PT providers (similar to the in-network doctor or hospital). Again, this is important because out-of-network providers will result in higher out-of-pocket expenses to you personally. As has been mentioned, most health insurance plans allow a specific number of physical therapy visits per calendar year. Look into this and be aware of it as you rehabilitate after your surgery. Make sure you share this information with your PT as well so that she can tailor your program to maximize the number of visits you are allowed. Monitoring this information will assure that you do not exceed the number of visits allowed. If you need additional physical therapy visits, understanding your benefit will help your providers appeal for additional services on your behalf.

Surgical Assistants

Here's an example of potential mishap. Let's say your surgeon utilizes a surgical assistant who does not participate with your health insurance plan. Because of this, you personally could be expected to pay for this service. This fee can be anywhere from a couple of hundred dollars to several thousand depending on the complexity of your surgery. Or, your surgeon may request that two surgical assistants be present at your surgery if it is especially complex. You will need to clear this possibility for two reasons—to determine whether they're covered under the plan, and if so, whether the plan cover them both—so be sure to ask your surgeon about the surgical assistant issue before committing to a course of action. Being engaged in the process prior to your surgery will prevent surprises and may also give you an opportunity to negotiate or pre-pay for services that you may not have been aware of until several months after your surgery.

Thinking Ahead

One thing to consider is that this is an elective procedure and, as such, you can take your time and get all of your ducks in a row before proceeding. Most of the larger employers offer their workers multiple insurance options and give them the opportunity to switch policies at least once a year. If you are anticipating the need for a joint replacement, you may want to temporarily (for the year you decide to have surgery) switch to a policy with a slightly higher premium in favor of a lower deductible, co-pay, coinsurance, or maximum out-of-pocket expense. This is an individual decision based on your resources but should be given some consideration. Once the joint replacement is successfully completed, you can move back to your higher deductible insurance package at the next opportunity if you wish.

Long and Short Term Disability

Another issue to consider is that of short and long term disability insurance. If your employer offers either short term and/or long term disability coverage, or you have an individual disability policy that provides compensation (or other benefits) when you're unable to work for an extended absence, you should review the plan documents or meet with your Human Resources representative prior to your anticipated surgery to discuss the coverage and the process of applying for benefits. While most conventional disability insurance claims don't begin until you're physically unable to work, you can submit the application for your disability benefits prior to a planned/scheduled surgery date. By doing so, you'll be able to assure that the initial application has been submitted in a timely manner. You will also be able to communicate with your surgeon's office staff the expectations for providing your disability carrier with follow-up information regarding your recovery. By anticipating these factors you can potentially eliminate lengthy delays with your initial disability payments, thus assuring that your benefits won't be interrupted or late due to a lack of progress reports from your surgeon.

Summary for Insurance Matters

This is a complex subject, and this chapter lays out the ground rules. Each surgeon's office has a point of contact regarding financial questions and can add detail and guidance to this picture for you. If you have any questions about insurance-related issues, speak to the office manager or financial officer before you schedule surgery so that you know exactly what you'll be spending.

If you address the issues presented in this chapter, you will be well informed on financial issues surrounding the surgery and will be better able to focus on the physical and emotional aspects of the surgery itself without distractions.

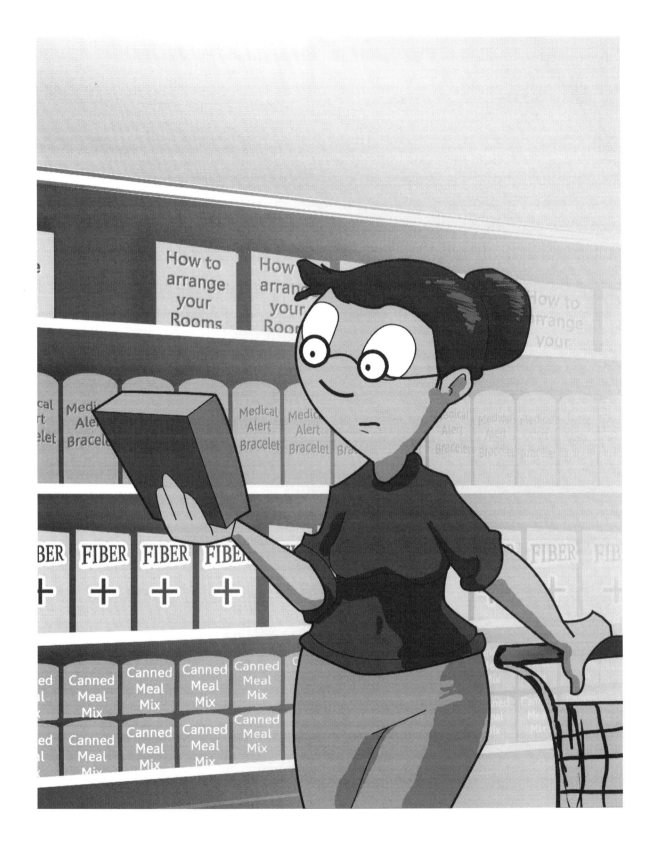

Checklists for the Home, Logistical Issues and the Hospital

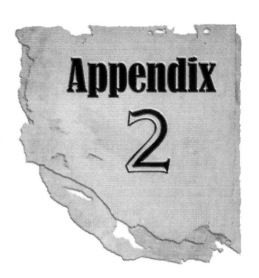

Appendix 2

by Dr. Hugate

Undergoing joint replacement surgery can be stressful for you personally and for your loved ones. Being prepared for surgery is the key to minimizing this stress. Once you have committed to undergoing joint replace surgery, the following checklist can be helpful in assisting with your preparation. With these preparations, you will have more time to focus on rehabilitation and healing after surgery.

Preparing Your Home

- ❑ Remove all throw rugs or loose rugs from your home as they are a falling hazard.
- ❑ Consider installing elevated toilet seats (especially if you have having your hip replaced) for use when you get home from surgery.
- ❑ Remove all extension cords from common walking paths in your home as they are a tripping hazard.
- ❑ Place night lights strategically throughout the house to light any common walking paths at night. (for example, to the bathroom or kitchen)

❑ Arrange your bed in an area of your home, such that the kitchen, bathroom, and bedroom are all on the same floor and in a place where you can get out safely in case of a fire. This will prevent you from having to go up and down stairs frequently for the first few weeks after surgery.

❑ Make sure you have a comfortable chair with a television nearby and perhaps a computer for use during the day.

❑ If you are having a hip replacement, remove any low chairs from your home as these can put you at risk for hip dislocation (popping out of joint). A chair is considered too low if, when you sit in it, your knees are above your hips.

❑ Make sure you have a few pairs of slip-on shoes. These are easier to use the in the first few weeks after joint replacement surgery.

❑ Purchase a "grabber/reacher" for help with picking up things off the floor. This may be difficult for the first few days/weeks after surgery. These can be purchased at most pharmacies.

❑ Purchase a long shoehorn. This will be helpful when getting your shoe on/off during the first few weeks after surgery. These can be purchased at most pharmacies.

❑ Have all of your laundry cleaned before surgery so you don't have to deal with laundry immediately when you get home.

❑ Have your vehicle(s) fueled up before you go to the hospital.

❑ Make sure you have a functional ice machine or access to ice when you get home so that you can apply ice to the wound if necessary.

❑ Repair any uneven surfaces or damaged floors as they will be tripping hazard.

❑ Consider buying a medical alert bracelet if you have significant medical problems.

❑ Make sure you have at least a 30 day supply of your usual home medications at home before you go in for surgery.

❑ Make sure you have a 30 day supply of stool softeners at home. You will need them after surgery because pain medications can cause constipation. Over-the-counter stool softener of your choice is fine.

❑ Consider preparing meals that can be frozen and reheated later when you are recovering so you don't have to cook for the first 2 weeks after surgery.

❑ Make sure you have a 30 day supply of you usual toiletries. (shampoo, soap, mouthwash, toothpaste, etc.) at home so that you aren't forced to go out and shop for them immediately after surgery

❑ Arrange your lawn care and snow removal for the 6 weeks following surgery.

❑ Arrange to have someone check on you twice a day (or have someone stay with you) when you get home from surgery for at least 2 weeks.

❑ If you have a pet, arrange pet care (i.e. kennel, grooming, walks, etc.).

❑ Make sure your cupboard is stocked with groceries for your return.

❑ Make sure you have a charged cell phone with " Hot Keys" to neighbors, 911, MD office, PCP office, local family/ friends and carry it with you all times when you get home.

❑ Consider installing handrails where needed (shower/tub/toilet)... especially if you are obese, have a history of falls, live alone, have balance problems, use crutches or a walker before surgery, or have osteoporosis (thin bones).

Other Logistical Issues to Consider

❑ Schedule your postoperative Physical Therapy appointment before you go in for surgery. The appointment should be scheduled for 5-6 days after your scheduled surgery. Please select a facility that is convenient for you and your family and make sure they accept your insurance.

❑ Arrange transportation to and from Physical Therapy after surgery. If you are on pain medications (and you will be) after surgery, you should not drive yourself.

❑ Arrange transportation to and from the hospital. Try to use a bigger vehicle with soft suspension if possible to make the trip more comfortable for you.

❑ Schedule and attend a 'Joint Replacement class' if offered by your surgeon.

❑ Ensure that you obtain a temporary handicapped parking permit from our office. This is good for 90 days from the date of issuance.

❑ Inform your employer that you will be out of work approximately 6 weeks (if your job is sedentary) or 3 months off (if your job is more labor intensive) following surgery. If you have disability forms/ FMLA paperwork that need to be completed, send them to your surgeon's office.

❑ Please see your dentist if you cavities or active infections of the teeth or gums at least 3 weeks prior to undergoing your surgery. Notify our office that you will be seeing your dentist and inform us as to the date of the appointment.

Items To Bring To The Hospital

❑ Glasses (not contacts) if necessary

❑ No-slip slippers/ slip on shoes (not lace up)

❑ 3 pairs of socks

❑ 3 pairs of underwear

❑ 1 set of street clothes

❑ 1 winter coat (if cold outside)

❑ Laptop computer

❑ Books and magazines of interest

❑ Deodorant/mouthwash

- ❑ House robe (not too long that you will trip on the tails)
- ❑ Hairbrush or comb (if necessary!)
- ❑ Empty stomach (do not have anything to eat or drink after midnight the night before)
- ❑ Insurance card
- ❑ Identification card
- ❑ A Grabber/Reacher
- ❑ A long shoe horn
- ❑ A folder for all your discharge papers/instructions
- ❑ Baby wipes
- ❑ Medical Power of Attorney or living will
- ❑ Any special small food items that you enjoy (unless you are on a special diet)
- ❑ IPOD or music player of choice with ear buds if you prefer to listen to music
- ❑ Only basic makeup if necessary
- ❑ A list of questions for your surgeon/ anesthesiologist to answer before surgery.

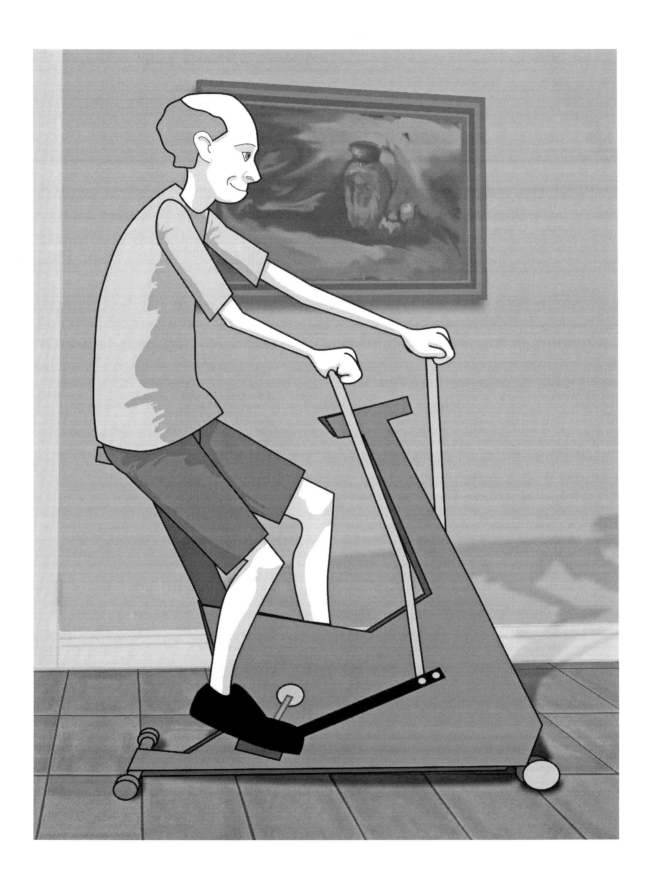

Exercises to Prepare for—or Rehabilitate from—Hip or Knee Replacement

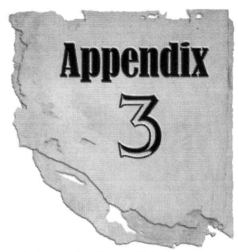

Appendix 3

by Dr. Hugate and Inger Brueckner

This section presents a few exercises which may be helpful in both preparing your body for joint replacement surgery and rehabilitation afterward. The goal is to improve strength and range of motion of your hip or knee. Of course, before beginning any course of exercises, *review them with both your doctor and physical therapist*. Remember—*it takes time, effort and dedication* to gain strength. Start slowly and work your way up to more repetitions and resistance. If you experience pain when doing any of these do not continue with the exercise.

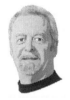

Holland's Comment: The adjoining cartoon shows a total knee replacement (TKR) patient riding his home exercise bike, complete with synchronized hand grips. In *Chapter 14, Physical Therapy for Hip and Knee Replacement Surgery*, Inger explained that after TKR she often includes an exercise bike in her treatment. The challenge is to bend the new knee enough to go over the top, then straight enough to go all the way around. After both of my TKR's this wasn't possible for me. So, my PT had me go back and forth (in each direction) as far as I could tolerate (exploring my limits on each attempt to pedal completely) while she carefully monitored and assisted.

Your progress after a TKR will only be noticeable by the week because daily changes are imperceptible. However, after time and diligent effort, it wasn't too long after surgery before I finally made it over the top and as time went by, it became easier and easier. Now, I'm back riding my real bicycle all the time.

Before your surgery, this kind of unit is great for strengthening your legs and gluteus muscles because it also strengthens your arms and shoulders. Remember, you'll need some "upper body strength" for moving yourself about on the hospital bed (i.e. when using the trapeze assembly we showed you in *Chapter 13, The Hospital Stay*).~*~

Straight Leg Raise Exercise

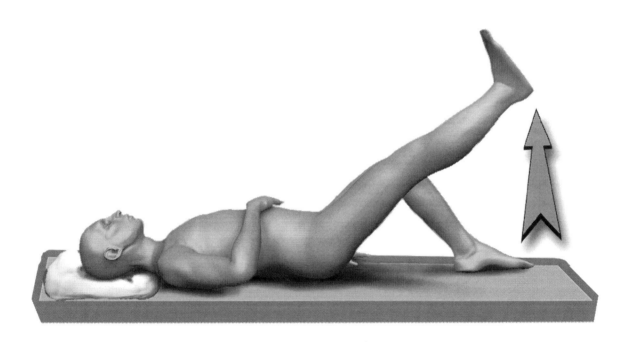

This is a simple exercise designed to strengthen your hip flexors and your quadriceps muscles after hip or knee replacement surgery.

Start by simply lying flat. Bend your non-operative knee about 45 degrees and plant your non-operative foot on the ground flat (to be used as a balance and push-off point). Keeping your operative knee straight, raise the leg by lifting from the hip as pictured above. Hold this position for 5 seconds and then allow the leg to lower slowly until it rests on the surface again.

Start with one set of 10 of these exercises without resistance. You may progress to up to 3 sets of 10 repetitions daily. As you gain strength, you may add light resistance (up to 5 lbs) by placing a weight strap around your ankle.

Hip Flexion Exercise

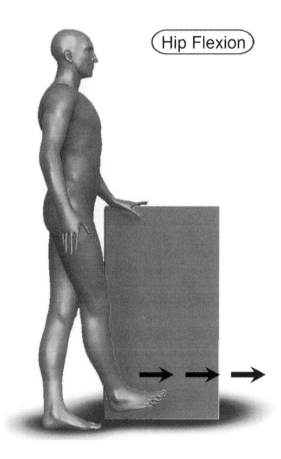

Hip Flexion

Another way to strengthen hip flexor muscles is the standing hip flexion exercise.

Start by standing upright with both feet firmly planted on the floor. Be sure to perform this exercise with a solid stable base nearby that you can place a hand on for balance. Now simply move the operative leg forward by flexing at the hip as shown. Keep your knee straight during this motion. Flex the hip up to about 40 degrees and hold that position for 5 seconds. Then relax the hips and let the leg slowly return to the standing position.

Start with one set of 10 of these exercises without resistance. You may progress to up to 3 sets of 10 repetitions daily. As you gain strength, you may add light resistance (up to 5 lbs) by placing a weight strap around your ankle.

Hip Abductor Exercise

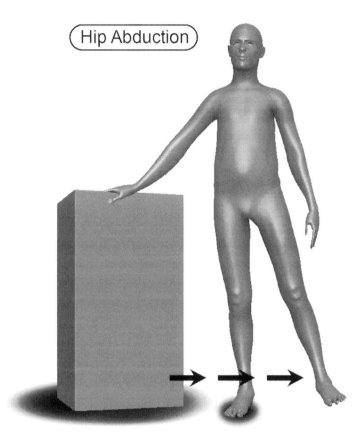

Hip abductor muscles can be especially weak after hip replacement surgery and may cause a limp. To strengthen the hip abductors use the "hip abduction" exercise. Stand with your hand on a stationary object to help with balance. Then move the operative leg outward (away from the midline) with the knee straight as shown. Bring the leg out to about a 30 degree angle with the body and hold that position for about 5 seconds. Then slowly allow the leg to return to its original position.

Start these exercises in the standing position as shown and perform one set of 10 repetitions. You can increase this to 3 sets of 10 repetitions as you are able. To add resistance, you can perform this exercise while lying on your side with the operative leg up. This adds gravity to the equation and therefore resistance. Once you are strong enough you can progress further by adding up to 5 lbs of ankle weight to either your standing or lying hip abduction exercises.

Clamshell Exercise

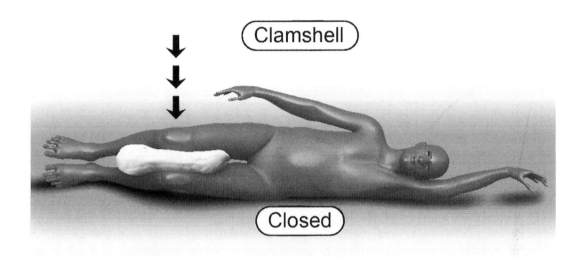

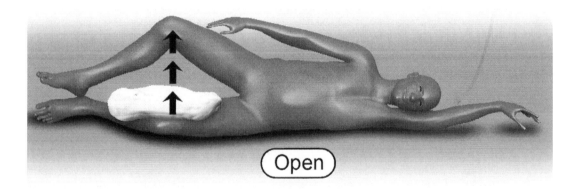

The "clamshell" exercise strengthens your hip rotator muscles and hip abductor muscles while increasing flexibility. Lying on your side with the operative leg up, place a pillow between your legs and don't let your legs cross. Bend your knees slightly. Then rotate and elevate your leg (as illustrated) to simulate the action of a clamshell opening and closing. Hold the up position for 5 seconds before slowly returning to the down position.

Start with one set of 10 repetitions of these exercises daily without resistance. You may progress to up to 3 sets of 10 repetitions daily. As you gain strength, you may add light resistance (up to 5 lbs) by placing a weight strap around or over your knee.

273

Hip Extension Exercise

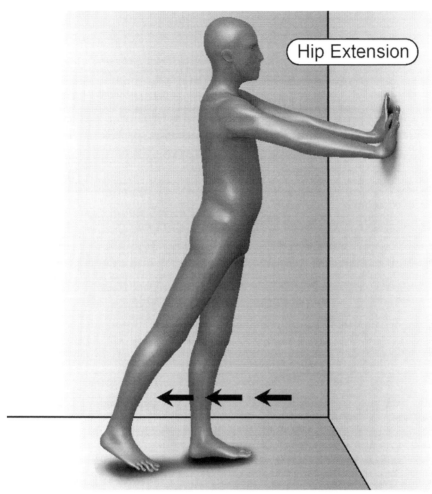

It's important for your gait, and when standing up, to have strong "hip extensor" (buttock) muscles. To exercise this group of muscles, stand in front of a wall and place both hands flat on the wall for balance. Then extend the operative leg by pushing the leg backwards while keeping the knee straight until the leg makes about a 30 degree angle with your body. Hold that position for 5 seconds and then slowly return to the standing position.

Start with one set of 10 repetitions of these exercises daily without resistance. You may progress to up to 3 sets of 10 repetitions daily. As you gain strength, you may add light resistance (up to 5 lbs) by placing weight strap around your ankle.

Supine Bridge Exercise

Supine Bridge

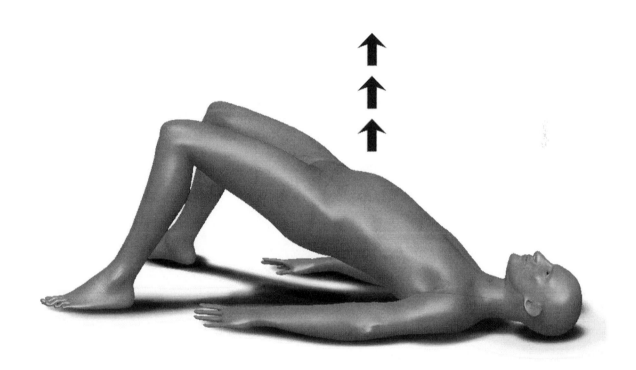

The "supine bridge" exercise is aimed mostly at strengthening the buttock (hip extensor) and hamstring muscles. While lying flat, bend your knees slightly and place your feet flat on the floor. Now arch your back and thrust your pelvis upwards to pick your bottom up off of the floor. Your arms should be planted flatly on the floor on either side and used as a support. Hold the up position for 5 seconds before returning your buttock slowly back to the surface.

Start with one set of 10 repetitions of these exercises daily without resistance. You may progress to up to 3 sets of 10 repetitions daily.

Glossary

A

abduction pillow A wedge-shaped pillow sometimes placed between the legs of a patient who has undergone hip replacement to prevent him from crossing his legs while he is lying down.

ABOS Abbreviation for the American Board of Orthopedic Surgery. This is the group in the United States responsible for certifying orthopedic surgeons.

acetabulum The bone that makes up the "socket" in the hip joint.

ACL Abbreviation for anterior cruciate ligament. See also —> **anterior cruciate ligament**.

activities of daily living Those activities that we perform routinely as part of our everyday lives, such as bathing, preparing meals, walking, and dressing.

ADL Abbreviation for activities of daily living. See also —> **activities of daily living.**

adult reconstruction The subspecialty within orthopedic surgery dealing with joint replacements.

anatomy The science of describing the parts of a body.

anesthesia A field of medicine which deals with eliminating or reducing pain.

anesthesiologist A physician who specializes in eliminating or reducing pain during surgical procedures. Some anesthesiologists also specialize in pain control of patients in the outpatient setting.

antagonists Two groups of muscles that work against one another across the same joint.

anterior Description of the position of an object in front of another object, or something positioned toward the front of the body.

anterior cruciate ligament A ligament within the knee which connects the tibia to the femur and stabilizes the knee joint. It prevents shifting of the two bones from front to back and also prevents excessive twisting of the knee during activities. Abbreviated as ACL.

anti-inflammatory A group of medications that are commonly taken in pill form to help reduce inflammation.

arthroscopy The insertion of small (pencil thickness) instruments into the joint space to directly examine the structures inside. Arthroscopic instruments can be used to remove or repair damaged cartilage that may be irritating the joint and to reconstruct ligaments if necessary.

articular cartilage The cartilage that is located on the ends of bones. This type of cartilage essentially "coats" the ends of the bone and acts to lubricate and cushion the joint.

arthrocentesis See also —> **aspiration**.

aspiration A procedure in which a needle is placed into a joint or space and the fluid within that joint or space is removed. Also known as arthrocentesis.

avascular necrosis A condition in which bone dies through interruption of its blood supply. This is common in the hips and may be caused by breaking the hip, heavy alcohol use, heavy medical steroid use, and blood clotting disorders, among other things. When the bone dies around the joint, it may collapse and cause arthritis and pain. Abbreviated as AVN.

AVN Abbreviation for avascular necrosis. See also —> **avascular necrosis**.

B

Baby Boomers Americans born between the years 1946 and 1964. These are mostly children of returning military service men and women who decided to start a family upon their return from overseas conflicts.

bilateral A structure that is present on both sides of the body.

bipolar Also known as a hemi-arthroplasty, this is a type of partial hip replacement in which only the "ball" of the hip joint is replaced; the cup is not replaced.

block room A special room within or next to the operating room used by anesthesiologists to perform a nerve block prior to having surgery performed.

C

cartilage A specialized type of tissue found within joints that cushions and lubricates the movements of that joint.

central nerve block A form of anesthesia in which the nerves are blocked by a numbing medication injected around the spine.

coinsurance The amount of money that you must pay out-of-pocket (in addition to what your insurance pays) for a service or visit to a provider.

compartments Distinct areas within the knee joint that may be susceptible to wear or arthritis. There are three compartments in the knee joint: the medial, lateral, and patello-femoral compartments.

compliance Following the instructions given to a patient by the medical treatment team.

condyles Rounded joint surfaces on the ends of long bones.

continuous passive motion A machine used to automatically move your knee through a prescribed range of motion at a prescribed speed. Abbreviated as CPM.

contracture The inability to fully straighten a joint.

corticosteroids A group of powerful anti-inflammatory medications.

CPM Acronym for continuous passive motion. See also —> **continuous passive motion**.

curriculum vitae A summary of a person's academic and work history. Similar to a résumé but used more commonly in academic professions. Abbreviated as CV.

CV Abbreviation for curriculum vitae. See also —> **curriculum vitae**.

D

deep venous thrombosis A blood clot that forms within the deep veins of an extremity. Abbreviated as DVT.

deductible The amount of money that you must pay out-of-pocket before your insurance begins paying a portion of your medical bill.

deformity Any deviation in the normal angulation, curvature, or length of an extremity.

drain A plastic or rubber tube that your surgeon may place in your wound during surgery to help evacuate any blood which may accumulate in your wound after surgery. This is typically removed a day or two after surgery.

dura The "sac" around the spinal cord and spinal nerves. This sac holds the spinal fluid which bathes the spinal cord and nerves in nutrients.

DVT Abbreviation for deep venous thrombus. See also —> **deep venous thrombus**.

E

elective surgery A non-emergency surgery in which you have time to gather information, ask questions, interview doctors, and discuss with friends and family members whether or not to have surgery.

epidural Short for epidural anesthesia. See also —> **epidural anesthesia**.

epidural anesthesia A type of anesthesia which uses a soft plastic catheter inserted just below the spinal cord outside the dural sac to numb the lower half of the body by blocking the nerve signals as they exit the spinal canal. Epidural catheters can be left in after surgery for a few days to provide extended pain relief.

expectations The beliefs a patient has about how her joint will work and what level of activity she will be able to return to after surgery.

extension The act of straightening a joint.

extensor mechanism The muscles and tendons responsible for straightening the knee.

F

fellowship Additional training that a physician may take after graduating from residency to gain extra expertise in a certain subspecialty field.

femur The thighbone.

femoral component The part of a knee (or hip) replacement that fits on the end of the femur.

femoral head The "ball" portion of the hip joint.

fibula The long, thin bone on the outer aspect of the leg that connects the knee to the ankle.

flexion The act of bending a joint.

fracture A break in the bone.

G

general anesthesia A form of anesthesia in which the patient is given medication that produces deep sleep, so much so that they require a breathing tube and ventilator machine during surgery.

H

hamstrings A group of muscles behind the thigh which bend the knee when they contract.

hemi-arthroplasty Also known as a bipolar. A partial hip replacement in which only the "ball" of the hip joint is replaced. The "socket" of the hip joint is not replaced.

hip precautions A set of rules which govern how you can move your hips after hip replacement surgery to prevent the hip from dislocating (popping out of joint). The hip precautions vary depending on what technique was used to install your hip and should be received from your operative surgeon only.

hospitalist A doctor (usually an internal medicine specialist) who attends to your medical needs while you are in the hospital after surgery.

hyaluronic acid A type of injectible lubricant that is used to reduce pain when injected into joints, most commonly used in the knee joint. This is a treatment step that is used before surgery to help get pain and inflammation in the joint under control. Abbreviated HA.

hyperextension Extending a joint beyond the fully straight position.

I

inflammation A biological response to tissue irritation. Inflammation usually manifests itself as pain, swelling, warmth, and sometimes redness.

inpatient Refers to a patient who is in the hospital.

instability Description that pertain to joints that are "sloppy" or "wobbly" in which the ligaments and tendons are loose and do not keep it stable.

internship The first year of training for doctors after medical school. Here physicians treat patients under the supervision of a senior surgeon.

intubation The act of placing a breathing tube in the windpipe for surgery. This is necessary for those who choose to go to sleep for surgery (undergo general anesthesia). It keeps the airway open so that fresh oxygen can flow to the lungs and protects the windpipe from obstruction.

invasive treatment Any treatment requiring that the skin be cut (or broken).

J

joint The anatomic structure where bones come together. Most joints have a capsule and ligaments that surround them and viscous fluid within them to help lubricate their movements. They also usually have cartilage which helps to cushion the ends of the bones as well.

k

kneecap See also —> **patella**

L

lateral Describes a structure that is further away from the midline of the body.

lateral collateral ligament A ligament on the outside of the knee that connects the femur to the fibula and keeps the knee from moving excessively from side to side. Abbreviated as LCL.

LCL Abbreviation for lateral collateral ligament. See also —> **lateral collateral ligament.**

ligament A tight band of tissue that connects one bone to another bone.

local anesthetic A medication which, when injected near a nerve, will block all pain transmission through that nerve.

M

MA Abbreviation for medical assistant. See also —> **medical assistant.**

manipulation under anesthesia A procedure performed rarely after knee replacement in order to break up scar tissue and regain range of motion. It generally consists of a patient going to sleep for a short time (usually only a few minutes) while the surgeon bends and straightens the knee to break up scar tissue.

MCL Abbreviation for medial collateral ligament. See also —> **medial collateral ligament.**

medial collateral ligament A ligament on the inside of the knee that connects the femur to the tibia and keeps the knee from moving excessively from side to side. Abbreviated as MCL.

mechanical symptoms Symptoms in a joint such as locking or catching.

medial A structure that is closer to the midline of the body.

medical assistant A member of the surgeon's office staff whose responsibilities may include greeting patients, triaging phone calls, helping arrange the surgeon's schedule, scheduling tests, gathering information, and scheduling surgeries. Abbreviated as MA.

meniscus A type of cartilage found in the knee, shaped like a 'C', that helps to cushion the knee joint and create a better fit between the flat tibial surface and the rounded femoral surface.

methicillin resistant staphylococcus aureus A type of bacteria that are resistant to certain antibiotics and can cause infection. Abbreviated as MRSA.

MRSA An acronym for methicillin resistant staphylococcus aureus. See also —> **methicillin resistant staphylococcus aureus.**

MUA Abbreviation for manipulation under anesthesia. See also —> **manipulation under anesthesia.**

muscle The tissues of the human body that contract to pull on tendons and move a joint.

N

narcotics A family of pain medications (example: morphine).

nerve block A type of anesthesia in which a specific nerve is numbed with medication to reduce or eliminate pain in a particular part of the body.

non-elective surgery Emergency surgery. There is limited (or no) time to ask questions, choose a surgeon, measure options, and so on.

non-invasive treatment A form of treatment that does not involve breaking the skin.

NP Abbreviation for nurse practitioner. See also —> **nurse practitioner**.

NSAIDS Abbreviation for nonsteroidal anti-inflammatories. See also —> **anti-inflammatory**.

nurse A medical professional who has expertise in caring for patients both in the hospital and in the outpatient setting. Nurses are compassionate caregivers who perform a broad range of vital tasks, such as coordinating patient care, delivering medications, and assessing the sick or injured. Nurses are the lifeblood of any hospital and are the front-line professionals in patient care.

nurse practitioner A medical professional (similar to a physician assistant) who practices under the supervision of a physician (or sometimes independently). Nurse practitioners usually have the authority to write orders in the hospital chart and write prescriptions. Sometimes they are referred to as "physician extenders" because they improve the doctor's ability to care for a higher volume of patients.

O

occupational therapist A type of therapist similar to a physical therapist whose goals are to teach patients to adapt to and successfully complete practical tasks (for example, getting dressed after surgery or injury). Although occupational therapists help teach patients to deal with all sorts of practical tasks, they tend to focus on those tasks involving the arms and hands. Abbreviated as OT.

orthopedic surgeon A surgeon who specializes in the treatment of injuries or diseases of the muscles, joints, and bones of the body.

osteoarthritis Also known as "wear and tear" arthritis, this is irritation of a joint due to injury to the cartilage. Osteoarthritis can result from years of degenerative changes or can occur after a joint is traumatically injured. Flare-ups of pain tend to progressively worsen in frequency and intensity over the years. There is no known cure. As with most medical conditions, osteoarthritis is caused by a combination of factors including lifestyle, weight, and genetics.

OT Abbreviation for occupational therapist. See also —> **occupational therapist**.

outpatient Refers to a patient who is not in the hospital.

P

PA Abbreviation for physician assistant. See also —> **Physician's Assistant**.

PACU Abbreviation for Post-Anesthesia Care Unit. Also known as the **Recovery Room**. See also —> **Recovery Room**.

Partial Knee replacement A type of knee replacement in which only a small portion of the knee is replaced rather than the entire joint. May be appropriate for those (rare) patients who suffer from arthritis in only one small area of the joint.

patella The small, disk-shaped bone that makes up the front of the knee joint. The patella rides in the trochlear groove of the knee and is connected to the quadriceps muscles above and the tibia below by way of the quadriceps tendon above and patellar ligament below. This bone provides the fulcrum for extending the knee. See also —> **kneecap**.

patello-femoral joint The space between the kneecap and the trochlea of the femur.

patello-femoral replacement A type of partial knee replacement in which only the parts of the patella-femoral joint (kneecap and trochlea) are replaced.

PE Abbreviation for pulmonary embolism. See also —> **pulmonary embolism**.

peripheral nerve block A form of anesthesia in which the major nerve near the site of your surgery is numbed by an injection of local anesthetic.

PCP Abbreviation for primary care provider. See also —> **primary care provider**.

physical therapist A licensed professional specializing in helping patients regain function after surgery, injury, or disease through the use of exercises, stretching, and education. Abbreviated as PT.

physical therapy The form of therapy that deals with helping patients regain function after surgery, injury, or disease through the use of exercises, stretching, and education.

physical therapy assistant A trained professional who works under the supervision of the physical therapist to help implement and administer physical therapy.

physician assistant A medical professional (similar to a nurse practitioner) who practices under the supervision of a physician (or sometimes independently). Physician assistants usually have the authority to write orders in the hospital chart and write prescriptions. Sometimes they are referred to as "physician extenders" because they improve the doctor's ability to care for a higher volume of patients.

physiology The science of describing how the parts of the body work.

poly Abbreviation for polyethylene. See also —> **polyethylene**.

polyethylene A type of strong and durable plastic used as a bearing surface in knee and hip replacement surgery due to its low wear characteristics and low friction.

posterior Refers to an object behind another object, or something located toward the back of the body.

posterior cruciate ligament This is an important ligament within the knee which connects the tibia to the femur and stabilizes the knee joint. It prevents shifting of the two bones from front to back and also prevents excessive twisting of the knee during activities. It crosses the anterior cruciate ligament within the knee.

primary care provider The medical professional (usually a family practitioner, internist, nurse practitioner, or physician assistant) whom you See also —> regularly for health maintenance, and who is responsible for coordinating your overall medical care. Abbreviated PCP.

PT Abbreviation for physical therapist. See also —> **physical therapist**.

PTA Abbreviation for physical therapy assistant. See also —> **physical therapy assistant**.

pulmonary embolism A blood clot which has lodged in the lungs and prevents blood from circulating through the lungs. Pulmonary embolisms can be fatal on rare occasion. Abbreviated PE.

pulse The palpable throbbing of a blood vessel when the heart beats.

Q

quadriceps The group of muscles in the front of the thigh that straightens the knee when they are contracted.

quadriceps tendon The tendon that connects the quadriceps muscles to the patella.

R

reacher A device used by joint replacement patients to help them pick objects up off of the floor without having to bend down too far.

rehabilitation The process of getting stronger and more functional after surgery or injury.

rehabilitation facility A facility that patients sometimes go to when they are discharged from the hospital after surgery or injury; usually for patients who are medically stable but not ready to return home from a function standpoint. The goal is to administer intensive physical therapy to the patient until she is ready to go home and live independently.

range of motion The distance through which a joint can move measured in degrees.

recovery room The room to which patients go immediately after surgery to recover from anesthesia before going to the floor. Also known as the Post Anesthesia Care Unit, or PACU.

regional anesthesia A form of anesthesia in which a particular part of the body is numbed by blocking the nerve that provides sensation there.

residency The step in the training of physicians that comes after medical school and internship. Here physicians treat patients under the supervision of a senior surgeon.

rheumatoid arthritis A form of arthritis, referred to as "autoimmune arthritis," in which the body "attacks" its own cartilage. This is the second most common form of arthritis following osteoarthritis.

revision joint replacement Sometimes referred to as RTKR (revision total knee replacement) or RTHR (revision total hip replacement), an operation in which some or all of the parts of a failed joint replacement are removed and replaced.

S

SA Abbreviation for surgical assistant. See also —> **surgical assistant**.

second opinion Another opinion from a qualified professional regarding the diagnosis and recommended treatment of a medical problem.

skilled nursing facility A nursing home.

spinal Abbreviation for spinal anesthesia. See also —> **spinal anesthesia**.

spinal anesthesia A type of central, regional anesthesia in which the nerves are blocked as they exit the spinal cord by injecting medication into the fluid that surrounds the spinal cord.

State Licensing Board The organization responsible for licensing and policing medical professionals within a given state.

steroids Abbreviation for corticosteroids. See also —> **corticosteroids**.

symmetrical Structures that are mirror images of one another.

synovial fluid Thick viscous fluid within a joint that acts to lubricate the movements of that joint.

synovial Joint Highly mobile joints (such as the hip and the knee) that have lubricating joint fluid held around the joint by a thick lining.

synovial membrane (or lining) The lining within a joint that produces and contains the joint fluid.

T

tendon A strong band of tissue that connects muscles to bones. Muscles contract and pull through tendons to move joints.

tibia The large lower leg bone that connects the knee to the ankle.

tibial component The part of a knee replacement that is placed on the tibia.

tibial tubercle A small bump on the front of the tibia just below the knee.

This is where the patellar ligament (extensor mechanism) inserts and pulls on the leg to straighten the knee.

THR Abbreviation for total hip replacement. See also —> **total hip replacement.**

TKR Abbreviation for total knee replacement. See also —> **total knee replacement**.

total hip replacement A surgical procedure in which the arthritic, painful hip joint is removed and replaced with a mechanical joint consisting of metal, plastic, and sometimes ceramic materials. Abbreviated as THR.

total knee replacement A surgical procedure in which the arthritic, painful knee joint is removed and replaced with a mechanical joint consisting of metal, plastic, and sometimes ceramic materials. Abbreviated as TKR.

tourniquet An inflatable cuff that is placed on an extremity to reduce the amount of blood flowing into that extremity (usually during surgery) to reduce the amount of blood loss.

transfusion Receiving blood or blood products through an IV. This can be either blood that you, yourself donated ("autotransfusion") or taken from a blood bank ("allotransfusion").

trochlea The "groove" in the front of the femur in which the kneecap rides.

U

unicondylar knee replacement A type of partial knee replacement in which only the medial or lateral compartment are replaced. The rest of the joint is not replaced.

V

viscosupplementation A type of joint injection that is used to add lubrication to the fluids of the joint.

Index

A

ABOS: 47-48

acetabulum: 36

ACL: 31 —> See Also *anterior cruciate ligament*

activities of daily living: 66, 190 —> See Also *ADLs*

ADLs: 67, 190 —> See Also *activities of daily living*

adult reconstruction: 48

anatomy: 28, 35, 40, 141, 154

anesthesia: 63, 64, 69, 75, 83-84, 129, 134, 138, 166-167, 174, 182, 183-184, 251

anesthesiologist: 71, 83, 107-115, 118, 121-125, 129-130, 132-133, 138, 139, 144, 147, 167

antagonists: 34

Anterior: 28

anterior cruciate ligament: 31 —> See Also *ACL*

anti-inflammatory: 17, 18, 72 —> See Also *NSAIDS*

Arthroscopy: 21

avascular necrosis: 21 —> See Also *AVN*

AVN: 21 —> See Also *avascular necrosis*

B

bilateral: 63-67

block room: 134

C

cartilage: 15, 16, 19-21, 29, 30, 32, 35, 36, 38, 72, 141

compartment: 32

Compliance: 57

condyle: 30, 32

continuous passive motion: 135, 166, 170 —> See Also *CPM*

corticosteroids: 18

T

V

Table of Figures

Table of Figures

Table of Figures

Credits and Contacts

RD Holland, PMP:
- Acquisitions
- Photos (except our contributor's and Dr. Hugate's photos)
- Photographic Processing
- Handbook Design and Layout
- Project Manager
- Business Manager
- Media Development
- Indexing
- Cross Referencing
- Cartoon Captions
- Figure Captioning

Ryan Counts, CGA:
- Handbook Cover
- Handbook Cover Art & Layout
- Chapter Covers
- Illustrations
- Drawings
- Cartoons

For inquiries, contact Mr. Robert Holland at:

robert@Roxytone.com

www.HipandKneeHandbook.com

Made in the USA
Lexington, KY
02 June 2013